BREASTFEEDING

A Parent's Guide

Eighth Edition

Amy Spangler, MN, RN, IBCLC

☐ Wait to introduce pacifier/bottel → 3-4 weeks → Don't introduce bottel
 - 8-10 times in 24 hrs / marbel stomach - ~~infant~~ Day 1 6 mL
 - day 3 walnut size stomach 26 mL
 - day 10 - egg size stomach 600 mL

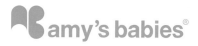
amy's babies®

Contributors
Doraine Bailey, MA, "Combining Breastfeeding and Working"
Rebecca F. Black, MS, RD/LD, IBCLC, "Eating for Two"
Karen Kerkhoff Gromada, MSN, RN, IBCLC, "Breastfeeding More Than One Baby"
Martha Hall, MSN, RN, IBCLC, and Sandra Jones, RD, MEd, IBCLC, "Breastfeeding Beyond the First Year"
Elizabeth Hormann, EdM, IBCLC, "Breastfeeding an Adopted or Previously Weaned Baby"
Dennis L. Spangler, MD, "Breastfeeding a Baby with a Family History of Allergic Disease"
Mary Rose Tully, MPH, IBCLC, "Breastfeeding a Premature Baby"

Production
Cover Design: thehappycorp global, thehappycorp.com, New York, New York, USA
Cover Photography: Doctor Jaeger, doctorjaeger.com, New York, New York, USA
Editing and Design: Carol Adams Rivera, MA, Health Communication Connection, healthcommunication.info, Vienna, Virginia, USA
Illustrations: Rick Powell, studiopowell.com, Montpelier, Vermont, USA
Printing: Specialty Lithographing Co., Cincinnati, Ohio, USA

12 11 10 09 08 07 06   2 3 4 5

ISBN 0-9729988-6-1

Library of Congress Catalog Card Number: 2005905323

To my sons

Matthew and Adam

my best teachers

Contents

Author's Notes

This book is designed so that each chapter provides complete information on the topic being discussed. As a result, some information is found in more than one chapter.

Throughout the book, in an effort to keep the text clear and easy to read, the baby is referred to as *he* or *him* when a personal pronoun is necessary. The terms *milk* and *breastmilk*, when used, refer to human milk.

Foreword

Breastfeeding is the most precious gift a mother can give her baby. Breastfeeding has numerous advantages for both infant and mother. A woman preparing for childbirth needs to think about how she is going to feed her baby before the baby arrives. After a discussion with her obstetrician or midwife and, of course, with her partner, a woman needs some help and reinforcement about her decision as she continues to think about it. Amy Spangler's BREASTFEEDING, *A Parent's Guide* provides the information necessary to make a comfortable decision, thoroughly reviewing all the questions parents have. No woman is born knowing how to breastfeed, and it is not a reflex that develops; she must learn. Learning how to breastfeed is well-described in this parent's guide. It can be read and reread when breastfeeding is underway. Amy has made it clear and simple with her illustrations and instructions. It is pleasant reading.

As breastfeeding is initiated, questions may arise about the infant, the breasts, the milk, or the mother. The author has anticipated these questions and provides clear, concise answers. The discussion about less common problems that may occur is extremely valuable. It helps the reader determine what to watch for and when to call either the mother's or the infant's physician.

The highly publicized problems with breastfeeding are extremely rare and have been traced back in each case to the mother's lack of information about simple problems and the failure to ask for help from her health care provider. This book will be a reliable guide for parents in recognizing problems early and seeking help appropriately.

The author is an experienced nurse and mother who knows all phases of the childbirth process. Furthermore, Amy is an educator as well and knows how to share information in a clear, concise, complete manner. This parent guide is an ideal source of information. Now in its eighth edition, it has been well-received by health care practitioners to supplement their patients' understanding of breastfeeding and provide an ongoing reference source about special situations. It is an excellent resource on both the art and the science of breastfeeding for parents.

Ruth A. Lawrence, MD
Professor of Pediatrics, Obstetrics, and Gynecology
University of Rochester School of Medicine and Dentistry
Rochester, New York

Preface

When I began teaching childbirth education classes almost 30 years ago, very few parents chose to breastfeed. But as knowledge of the benefits of breastfeeding and the consequences of not breastfeeding has increased, so too has the choice to breastfeed.

I taught my first breastfeeding class in 1984 (I won't tell you how old I was!). To encourage attendance, classes were held in the evening and were provided free of charge. Knowing that many parents had never seen a baby breastfeed, breastfeeding mothers, fathers, and babies, eager to share their new skill, were invited to each class. I wanted parents to see (and believe) that every parent (with few exceptions) can breastfeed.

In 1985, with the encouragement of the many parents I had taught, I wrote the first edition of *BREASTFEEDING, A Parent's Guide.* I understood that parents wanted a book that was clear, concise, and easy to read—not a dictionary, not an encyclopedia, not a medical textbook, but a practical guide to breastfeeding.

With the completion of this eighth edition, I marvel at how much I have learned since I wrote the first edition. While the art of breastfeeding has endured over centuries, knowledge of the science of breastfeeding has increased greatly in recent years. Today, parents choosing to breastfeed face special challenges and seek realistic solutions. *BREASTFEEDING, A Parent's Guide* acknowledges those challenges, and provides practical advice and down-to-earth solutions.

Breastfeeding is a learned skill, like riding a bicycle, only this bicycle is built for two! While many mothers and babies breastfeed without difficulty, others require help, especially in the early weeks. Fortunately, the breastfeeding problems featured in the media are rare, but serve to remind parents and professionals that breastfeeding is a skill that requires not only patience and persistence but knowledge and support. While *BREASTFEEDING, A Parent's Guide* provides the knowledge parents need to breastfeed, parents often look to family, friends, and health care providers for support. So keep this book handy and don't hesitate to ask your doctor, midwife, lactation consultant, or nurse for help.

I am forever grateful to those parents who have shared with me one of the most intimate experiences of their lives, breastfeeding their baby. I hope that they have learned as much from me as I have learned from them.

Amy Spangler

Introduction

One of the most important choices you will need to make as new
parents is whether to breastfeed or bottle-feed your baby. While the
benefits of breastfeeding for both mother and baby are quite clear, the
choice to breastfeed, as well as breastfeeding success, requires knowledge and support. A clear understanding of how the process works and
knowledge of how to manage problems that can occur are helpful. But
encouragement and support seem to be the keys to success.

Most physicians and parents agree that breastfeeding is the best
method of infant feeding, yet many parents choose to bottle-feed their
babies or stop breastfeeding after a brief period of time. Frequently
their choice is based upon too little information, incorrect information,
or too little support. Amy Spangler's *BREASTFEEDING, A Parent's Guide*
is a wonderful resource for breastfeeding parents. It is a practical step-
by-step guide to breastfeeding. It deals honestly and directly with the
advantages as well as the concerns. The review of milk production is
simple, yet complete and gives the reader a clear understanding of this
natural process. The suggestions for beginning to breastfeed provide
recommendations that can be changed to meet the needs of each
mother and baby. The discussions of possible problems, special situations, and common questions answer nearly all of the concerns
expressed by new parents.

The information found throughout this book, appropriate medical
advice, and encouragement and support from someone they trust will
help those parents who choose to breastfeed, breastfeed successfully
and encourage those who are undecided to seriously consider breastfeeding.

Richard Bucciarelli, MD
Professor of Pediatrics
Associate Chairman, Department of Pediatrics
Chief, Division of Neonatology
University of Florida
Gainesville, Florida

1 Benefits of Breastfeeding

Whether you plan to breastfeed or are unsure, you need to know how breastfeeding helps both you and your baby!

Benefits to You

Health

- Women who breastfeed have less risk of prolonged or heavy vaginal bleeding after their babies are born.

- Breastfeeding helps the uterus return to its normal size.

- Women who breastfeed lose their pregnancy weight more easily than women who formula-feed.

- Breastfeeding reduces the risk of breast, uterine, and ovarian cancer.

- Breastfeeding improves bone thickness and reduces the risk of osteoporosis and hip fractures in older women.

Social

- Breastfeeding requires no mixing, measuring, or clean-up, which makes nighttime feedings quick and easy.

- Breasts and babies are portable. Travel can be simple. With a little practice, mothers can breastfeed anywhere. Mothers who are shy or easily embarrassed might want to choose a quiet place where they will not be disturbed.

- Breastmilk is always available and at just the right temperature! There is no need to worry about storage or refrigeration. This is very important for mothers and babies in emergency situations where food supplies are limited or spoil easily.

Emotional

- Breastfeeding promotes a special relationship between a mother and her child, a closeness that comes with time and touch, a bond that lasts forever.

- Breastfeeding gives mothers a chance to rest during the day, something every new mother needs.

- With one hand free, a breastfeeding mother can share her time and attention with other children or take care of personal needs.

Economic

- Parents who breastfeed save an average of $1,000 in infant feeding costs during the first year.

- Breastfed babies have fewer illnesses, doctor visits, and hospital stays. So parents who breastfeed save an average of $400 in health care costs during the first year.

- Breastfed babies are healthier, even if they are in child care. So their parents who work outside the home miss fewer days of work and lose less income.

Environmental

- Breastmilk saves energy. No gas, oil, coal, or electricity is needed to make breastmilk. All you need is a breast, a baby, and a brain!

- Breastfeeding protects the environment. The only by-products are healthy mothers and babies!

- Breastmilk comes pre-packaged in individual servings. There's no need for glass or plastic containers.

Benefits to Your Baby

Health

- Human milk is the perfect food for your baby. It contains more than 200 nutrients plus special factors that protect your baby's health.

- Human milk changes to meet the needs of a growing baby, something formula cannot do.

- Human milk is easy to digest, so breastfed babies have less gas, colic, and spitting up.

- Breastfed babies have less diarrhea and constipation.

- Breastfed babies are less likely to develop chronic bowel diseases including ulcerative colitis, Crohn's disease, and celiac disease.

- Breastfed babies have fewer urinary tract infections.

- Breastfed babies have fewer respiratory infections and ear infections.

- Breastfeeding lowers the risk of asthma, colic, food allergy, and eczema in infants with a family history of allergic disease.

- Breastfeeding makes vaccines work better.

- Breastfed babies are less likely to develop insulin-dependent diabetes mellitus.

- Breastfed babies are less likely to develop some childhood cancers, including leukemia and lymphoma.

- Breastfed babies are less likely to become obese children.

- Breastfeeding promotes nervous system development and increases intelligence quotient (IQ).

- Breastfeeding may reduce the risk of sudden infant death syndrome (SIDS), the leading cause of death in babies between 1 month and 1 year of age.

Emotional

- Breastfeeding gives babies a chance to touch, to smell, to hear, to see, to taste, to know their mothers from the first moment of birth.

Common Concerns

Breastfeeding is best for you and your baby. But some parts of breast-feeding may seem bothersome at first. Be patient—the parts that are annoying are usually short-lived!

- **"Will I be able to come and go easily?"**
  Frequent breastfeedings may limit your freedom for the first 4–6 weeks while you are increasing your milk supply and learning to breastfeed. *But this gives you a chance to rest and to get to know your baby.*

- **"How can I keep my breasts from leaking?"**
  Leaking often occurs in the early weeks when babies are feeding at irregular times. *But leaking can be managed easily and is a sign of good milk production and milk release.*

- **"Will breastfeeding be painful?"**
  Breastfeeding can be painful at the beginning of a feeding when your baby first latches on to the breast. *But the pain should last only a few seconds if your baby is positioned correctly on the breast and has a good, deep latch.*

- **"How can I tell if my baby is getting enough to eat?"**
  The amount of milk taken at each feeding cannot be measured. *But you can be sure that your baby is getting enough to eat if he has frequent, runny, yellow stools (bowel movements).*

- **"Will every diaper be a poopy diaper?"**
  Breastfed babies stool frequently. *But their stools have little or no odor, so diapering is more pleasant. This is particularly important for fathers, who often have diaper duty!*

- **"When will my baby sleep through the night?"**
  Breastfed babies normally eat 8–12 times in each 24 hours and may not sleep through the night for many weeks or months. *But the same is true of many formula-fed babies.*

- **"Do I have to follow a special diet?"**
  You will want to limit your intake of alcohol and caffeine. *But you do not need to follow a special diet while breastfeeding, unless you have a family history of allergic disease or find that certain foods make your baby fussy.*

■ **"Can I take birth control pills while I am breastfeeding?"**
Birth control pills that contain estrogen can decrease your milk supply and should be avoided. But pills that contain only progesterone are thought to be safe. You should wait until your milk supply is well established (at least 6 weeks) before you start taking even progesterone-only pills (Figure 1). If you take progesterone-only pills and your milk supply decreases, talk to your health care provider right away. If you breastfeed fully (exclusively or almost exclusively), you can space your children naturally using the Lactational Amenorrhea Method (LAM). For LAM to be effective, the following conditions must apply:

• You have had no menstrual period (monthly bleeding) since the birth of your baby.

• You breastfeed fully, giving juice, formula, or water rarely.

• Your baby breastfeeds at least every 4–6 hours during the day and at night.

• Your baby is less than 6 months of age.

Many other birth control options are available as well. (See "If I breastfeed, can I still get pregnant?" p. 165.)

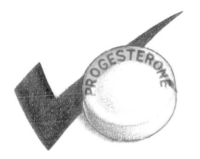 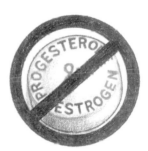

Figure 1
Mothers who breastfeed should not take birth control pills that contain *estrogen*. However, birth control pills that contain *only progesterone* are thought to be safe.

More Is Better!

Any amount of breastmilk is good for your baby. But research has shown that babies breastfed exclusively for 6 months are healthier—not just in infancy but for many years to come—than babies fed infant formula or a combination of formula and breastmilk. Your baby is worth the time and effort. Breastfeeding is easier than you think!

2 Understanding Milk Production

All You Need Is a Breast, a Baby, and a Brain!

The human breast is an amazing organ that changes to meet the needs of your baby. You may find it easier to breastfeed if you know the parts of the breast and understand how each part works during *lactation* (milk production) (Figure 2).

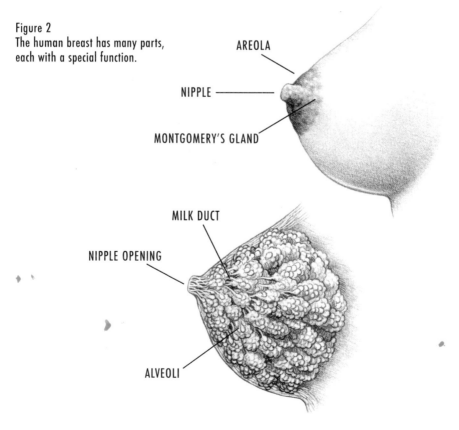

Figure 2
The human breast has many parts, each with a special function.

AREOLA

NIPPLE

MONTGOMERY'S GLAND

MILK DUCT

NIPPLE OPENING

ALVEOLI

For effective breastfeeding to take place, three things must happen: milk production, milk release, and milk transfer. For these three things to happen, all you need is a breast, a baby, and a brain (Figure 3).

Figure 3
To breastfeed, all you need is a breast, a baby, and a brain.

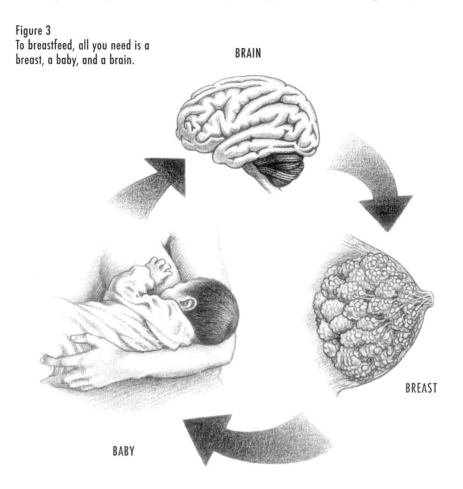

BRAIN

BREAST

BABY

When your baby begins to breastfeed, a message is sent to your brain. Your brain receives the message and sends a signal to the *pituitary gland*, a small group of cells attached to the base of the brain. The pituitary gland receives the signal and releases two hormones, *prolactin* and *oxytocin*. Prolactin tells your breast to make milk (milk production). Oxytocin tells your breast to release milk (milk release). Your baby then removes milk from your breast through breastfeeding (milk transfer) (Figure 4). The more milk your baby takes, the more milk you make!

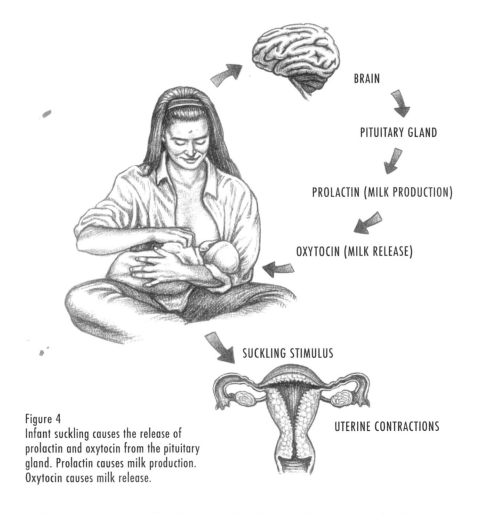

BRAIN

PITUITARY GLAND

PROLACTIN (MILK PRODUCTION)

OXYTOCIN (MILK RELEASE)

SUCKLING STIMULUS

UTERINE CONTRACTIONS

Figure 4
Infant suckling causes the release of
prolactin and oxytocin from the pituitary
gland. Prolactin causes milk production.
Oxytocin causes milk release.

Milk production, milk release, and milk transfer are described in more
detail below.

Milk Production

Milk is produced in the *alveoli,* grape-like sacs located deep inside the
breast (Figure 5). There are two types of cells in the alveoli—*secretory
cells* and *myoepithelial cells.* Secretory cells change fat and protein into
milk. Myoepithelial cells contract and move milk from the alveoli into
the *milk ducts.*

Milk production begins during pregnancy. Only a small amount of milk is
produced during pregnancy because of the presence of two hormones,

progesterone and *estrogen.* Progesterone and estrogen inhibit the release of prolactin and the production of milk during pregnancy. Progesterone and estrogen are produced by the *placenta.* The placenta is an organ that grows inside the *uterus* during pregnancy and transfers nutrients to your baby.

After your baby is born, the placenta is removed and progesterone and estrogen levels fall. Prolactin levels then rise, causing an increase in milk production. The increase in prolactin levels and milk production happens over a period of 3–5 days. If part of the placenta is left in the uterus after birth, milk production can be delayed until the placenta is removed.

Breastfeeding should begin as soon as possible after birth—ideally within the first hour. The amount of milk you produce depends on the amount of milk you remove from the breasts. Early, frequent breast-feedings (at least 8–12 feedings in each 24-hour period) will usually produce a good supply of milk.

Prolactin levels increase twofold each time your baby breastfeeds. This increase is thought to have a relaxing effect on you and your baby.

Figure 5
Milk production takes place in the alveoli, grape-like clusters of cells located inside the breast.

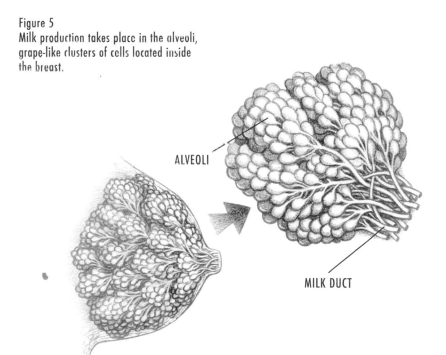

ALVEOLI

MILK DUCT

Milk Release

When your baby begins to breastfeed, the following events occur:

- Infant suckling signals the nerves inside the nipple to send a message to the brain—"Hungry baby!"

- The brain receives the message and signals the pituitary gland to release prolactin and oxytocin.

- Prolactin causes cells in the alveoli to make milk as described above.

- Oxytocin causes cells in the alveoli to contract. These contractions move milk from the alveoli into the milk ducts.

- Oxytocin also causes milk to be released through the nipple openings.

The flow of milk through the breast is called the *let-down reflex* or *milk-ejection reflex*. It may take several seconds or several minutes for the release of milk to occur. It may also take several days or weeks for the let-down reflex to develop fully.

Factors that can affect milk release include:

- embarrassment
- lack of confidence
- lack of encouragement and support
- pain
- stress
- tiredness

Milk Transfer (Removal)

Milk transfer is essential to effective breastfeeding. Some babies breast-feed often (8–12 times in each 24 hours) but do not transfer (remove) milk from the breast.

Correct positioning of your baby *at* and *on* the breast is the key to milk transfer (Figure 6). When your baby is positioned correctly *at* the breast, his chin, chest, and knees face the breast. When your baby is positioned correctly *on* the breast, his mouth is opened wide—as if he is yawning—and is filled with breast.

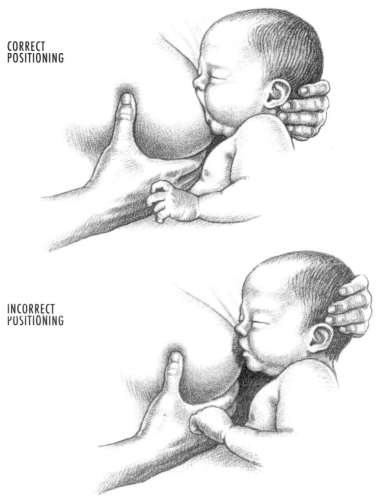

CORRECT
POSITIONING

INCORRECT
POSITIONING

Figure 6
When your baby is positioned correctly, his chin, chest, and knees face the breast and his mouth is opened wide. Your hand is below your baby's ears.

When a let-down reflex occurs, newly produced milk flows through the milk ducts. When your baby is positioned correctly on the breast, the milk ducts are drawn into your baby's mouth. With a wave-like movement of your baby's tongue, the milk ducts are compressed between the roof of the mouth above and the tongue below. The action of the tongue, beginning at the tip, moves milk through the ducts and out of the openings in the nipple (Figure 7).

When enough milk collects in your baby's mouth, a swallow occurs. Hearing or seeing your baby swallow is one sign of milk transfer. You may also see milk leaking from one breast while your baby breastfeeds from the opposite breast.

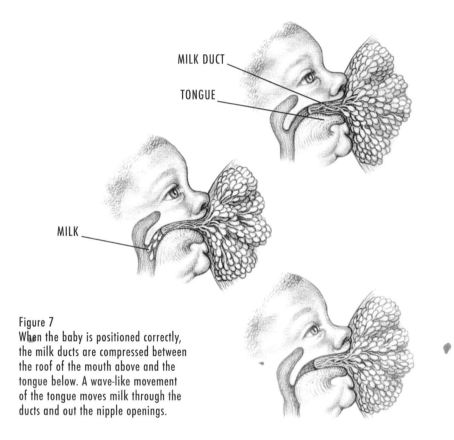

MILK DUCT

TONGUE

MILK

Figure 7
When the baby is positioned correctly, the milk ducts are compressed between the roof of the mouth above and the tongue below. A wave-like movement of the tongue moves milk through the ducts and out the nipple openings.

Maintaining a Milk Supply

The signal for continued milk production is the removal of milk from the breast through breastfeeding (infant suckling) or breast expression. Infant suckling causes a sudden increase in the level of prolactin. Prolactin plays an important role in maintaining milk production, but it does not affect milk volume. The amount of milk you make depends on the amount of milk your baby removes from the breast. This is the process of supply and demand. The more milk your baby removes from the breast, the more milk you will make.

When you delay or skip feedings and milk stays in the breast, the milk causes an increase in pressure. This pressure slows the flow of blood to the alveoli and causes a decrease in milk production. As long as your baby continues to breastfeed, you will continue to make milk. But if you limit the amount of breastfeeding by following a rigid feeding schedule or giving your baby water or formula supplements or a pacifier, your milk supply will decrease.

Types of Human Milk

There are three types of human milk: *colostrum*, transitional milk, and mature milk. Although each contains similar nutrients, they vary in content and volume. From 0 to 5 days after birth, colostrum is produced; from 5 to 10 days, transitional milk is produced; and after 10 days, mature milk is produced. The change from colostrum to mature milk is gradual and may occur unnoticed. The rate of change depends on how early and often your baby breastfeeds.

Colostrum

Colostrum is a fluid that can be thick and yellow or clear and runny. It is present during the last months of pregnancy and the first days after birth. Most mothers produce 1–3 ounces (30–90 ml) of colostrum each day. Colostrum is high in protein, low in fat, and rich in *antibodies* that protect your baby from infection. Colostrum also causes your baby's bowels to move early and often.

Transitional Milk

The content and volume of transitional milk change gradually over a period of 5 to 10 days. The rate of change is often slower in first-time mothers. If you have had a prior pregnancy or have breastfed before, mature milk may appear sooner. The amount of sugar, fat, and calories increases, while the amount of protein and antibodies decreases, until the levels for mature milk are reached.

Mature Milk

Mature milk has two parts, *hindmilk* and *foremilk*. Foremilk or *first milk* is low in protein, fat, and calories, giving it a thin, runny appearance. Hindmilk or *behind milk* is high in protein, fat, and calories, giving it a thick, creamy appearance (Figure 8). Hindmilk contains the fat and calories your baby needs to grow well.

Human milk changes to meet the needs of your baby, something formula cannot do. Human milk contains more than 200 substances. It is the perfect "fast food"—readily available and nutritious! The nutrients in human milk change from the beginning to the end of a feeding, from morning to night, from month to month, from mother to mother, and even from breast to breast! Although a mother's diet or health can have an effect on the nutrients in her milk, mothers on restricted diets and mothers who are poorly nourished are still encouraged to breastfeed.

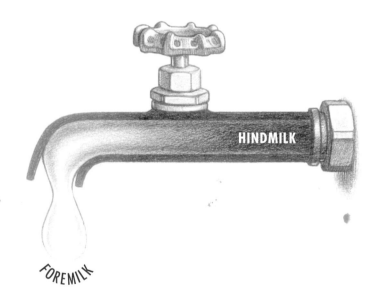

Figure 8
Foremilk is obtained at the beginning of a feeding, and hindmilk is obtained at the end of a feeding. Hindmilk contains more of the fat and calories babies need to grow. If you limit the length of breastfeedings, babies get little or no hindmilk.

3 Getting Ready to Breastfeed

Get Ready. Get Set. Go!

The best time to learn all that you can about breastfeeding is before your baby is born. Planning ahead will help you reduce the risk of problems and find solutions quickly if problems do occur. The more knowledge you have about breastfeeding, the easier breastfeeding will be once your baby arrives.

Caring for Your Breasts

Montgomery's glands, small pimple-like bumps in the darker part of your breast, produce an oily material that keeps your nipples clean and moist (Figure 2, p. 6). So no special care is needed before (or after) your baby is born. Simply wash your breasts with mild soap and water when you shower or bathe, and avoid the use of creams, lotions, and oils (Figure 9).

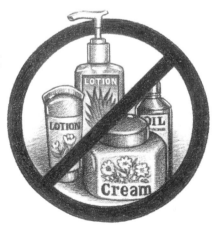

Figure 9
Avoid the use of creams, lotions, and oils on your breasts.

Nipple exercises or other types of nipple preparation should be avoided. These include nipple rolling or pulling, rubbing your nipples with a towel or washcloth, hand expression, or breast pumping. Any form of nipple stimulation can cause uterine contractions and can lead to premature labor. It is important to remember that nipple preparation does not prevent the tenderness and pain that can occur when you first begin to breastfeed. Positioning your baby correctly on the breast is the best way to prevent pain and avoid nipple damage.

During pregnancy the breasts often get fuller, the *areola* darkens, the Montgomery's glands enlarge, and a small amount of colostrum may drip from the nipples. Some women experience no breast changes, yet they still produce an ample supply of milk. If your breasts show no signs of change during pregnancy, let your health care provider know. Together you can ensure that your baby will get enough to eat.

Choosing Breastfeeding Supplies

Maternity shops, baby stores, and lactation centers offer a wide variety of breastfeeding supplies, including nursing bras, breast pads, nursing pillows, nursing clothes, breast creams, and breast pumps. Only three items are essential—a baby, a breast, and a brain! So before you buy items advertised as "essential," be sure the added convenience justifies the cost. For example, stretchy cotton T-shirts or blouses that button up the front offer easy access to the breast and can be a lot less expensive than nursing clothes. One of the many benefits of breastfeeding is cost savings. So before you stock up on supplies, consider the following.

Nursing Bras

You do not need to wear a bra during pregnancy or while breastfeeding. If you prefer to wear a bra, you may find nursing bras handy. A nursing bra has flaps that open over each breast, allowing you to breastfeed your baby without removing the entire bra. Nursing bras hold breast pads in place and can reduce leaking from the opposite breast during feedings.

Nursing bras can be purchased at maternity stores or lactation centers. For a proper fit, wait until the last weeks of your pregnancy. You may find it helpful to talk with a professional who is skilled at bra fitting. Choose comfortable bras with cotton cups, adjustable straps, and simple flap fasteners. Avoid bras with underwires or bras that are too tight or bind, making it difficult to remove milk from all parts of the breast. If you prefer a bra with underwires, remove the bra for one or two feedings during the day and at night. Comfortable "sleeping bras" can be worn at night to hold breast pads in place should leaking occur.

Breast Pads

Breast pads are used to protect clothes from leaking milk. Breast pads come in all shapes and sizes and are usually made from cotton or wool. Some pads are meant to be used only once, while others can be washed and used over and over again. Breast pads can be thick or thin. Thin pads can be less visible under clothing, but they may need to be changed more often. Remember to change pads frequently, and avoid pads with waterproof liners that trap wetness against the skin.

Nursing Clothes

You do not need to wear special clothes to breastfeed your baby, but some mothers find nursing tops and nightgowns convenient. Nursing clothes have openings over the breasts that are hidden in folds of fabric. The openings allow you to breastfeed your baby while keeping your clothes in place. Nursing clothes can make it easier to breastfeed discreetly in public, but the extra cloth can be bulky as well, so you may want to try different styles.

Meeting Special Needs

Many women worry that the size or shape of their breasts will affect their ability to produce milk. Breast size and shape are determined mainly by fat deposits. Though fat deposits protect the milk-producing cells in your breasts, they do not affect your ability to produce milk.

Nipple size and shape can make breastfeeding easier or harder for some babies. But most babies will learn to breastfeed on their mother's breasts if given the opportunity. All it takes is practice! The Pinch Test (Figure 10) can help you decide if your nipples are normal, flat, or inverted (Figure 11).

- Place your thumb and first finger at the base of the nipple near the edge of the areola.

- Press your thumb and finger together.

- A normal nipple will protrude or come out.

- A flat or inverted nipple will retract or sink in. (Truly inverted nipples are rare.)

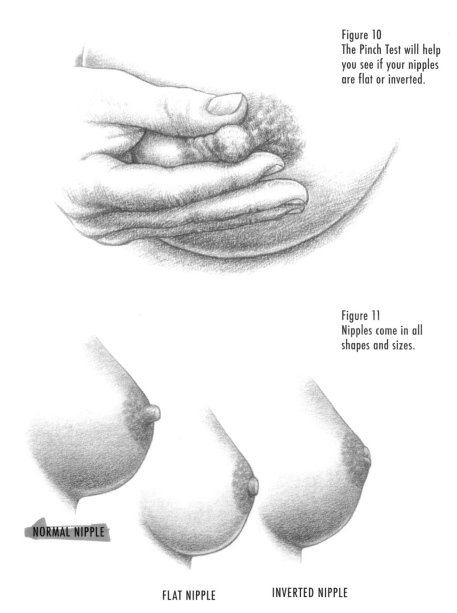

Figure 10
The Pinch Test will help you see if your nipples are flat or inverted.

Figure 11
Nipples come in all shapes and sizes.

NORMAL NIPPLE

FLAT NIPPLE   INVERTED NIPPLE

If you are concerned about the size or shape of your nipples, talk with your health care provider early in your pregnancy.

If your nipples are flat or inverted and your baby has trouble breast-feeding, you may find a breast pump helpful (Figure 12). You can use the pump before each breastfeeding to gently pull your nipple out. (See "Beginning to Breastfeed," p. 27.)

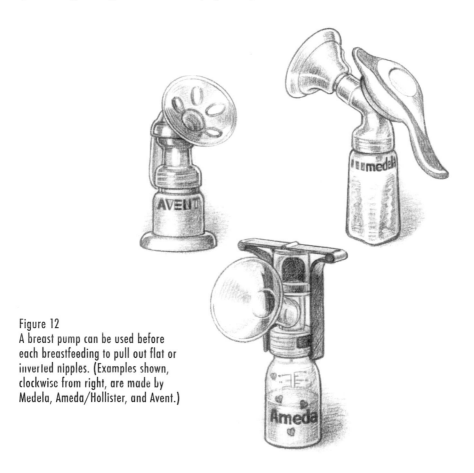

Figure 12
A breast pump can be used before each breastfeeding to pull out flat or inverted nipples. (Examples shown, clockwise from right, are made by Medela, Ameda/Hollister, and Avent.)

Breast Shells

Although some women choose to wear breast shells during pregnancy to treat flat or inverted nipples, research shows that breast shells are seldom helpful and may actually do more harm than good. In addition, some women find breast shells painful or embarrassing. You may prefer to wait until after your baby's birth to see if he has difficulty breastfeeding. Talk with your health care provider before you make a decision.

Nipple Shields

A nipple shield is a device that can be used in special situations to aid attachment, support milk transfer, and maintain breastfeeding (Figure 13). Babies who might benefit from the use of a nipple shield include premature babies who are unable to maintain a latch, babies who are accustomed to a bottle nipple and refuse to breastfeed, and babies of mothers with flat or inverted nipples. A nipple shield can be used at the start of a feeding to encourage your baby to latch on, and can then be removed after your baby begins to suckle and swallow. A nipple shield can also be used throughout the feeding.

There are different types of nipple shields, and some are more effective than others. A thick rubber (latex) shield is more likely to interfere with milk transfer than an ultra-thin silicone shield. All nipple shields are intended for short-term use until the breastfeeding problem is solved. Check with your health care provider before using a nipple shield. If you decide to use a nipple shield, check your baby's weight often (at least weekly) so you can be sure that he is getting enough to eat.

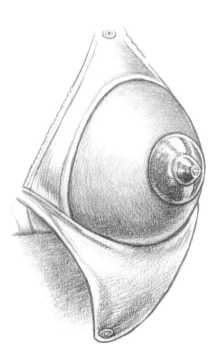
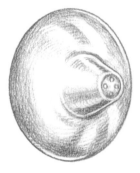

Figure 13
Nipple shields can make latch-on easier when
a mother has a flat or inverted nipple.
However, a nipple shield can limit milk
production, milk release, and milk transfer.

Planning Ahead

Caring for a new baby takes time, no matter how you choose to feed your baby. So try to complete as many tasks as possible before your baby is born.

- Prepare a space for your baby. This can be a separate room (a nursery) or part of a room.

- Get a crib or bassinet and a car seat that meet safety standards.

- Take infant CPR/first aid and baby care classes.

- Choose a health care provider for your baby.

- Make a list of nearby lactation support services.

- Prepare and freeze meals for later use.

- Pay household bills early.

- Write thank-you notes for baby gifts already received.

- Address and stamp envelopes if you plan to send birth announcements.

- Complete all work-related projects.

- Clean and organize your apartment or home.

- Last but not least, spend time with your partner. Once your baby arrives, time will be in short supply!

4 Beginning to Breastfeed

Ready or Not, Here He Comes!

You know how the breast makes milk. Now you need to learn how to get the milk into your baby. With the excitement of your baby's birth, it is easy to forget what you have learned. So you might want to keep this book handy and take it to the hospital with you.

Your Baby's First Breastfeeding

- **Breastfeed as soon as possible after birth**. If both you and your baby are healthy, you should begin breastfeeding within the first hour, when your baby is likely to be quiet and alert. This first breastfeeding is a learning experience for you and your baby, so relax and enjoy this time together. Many babies are content to lick, taste, smell, and snuggle, safe and warm against their mother's breast. Others will latch on and suckle if given the chance. Every baby is different.

- **Keep your baby with you day and night**. Mothers and babies should stay together (sharing a room 24 hours a day) whenever possible. Sharing a room gives you and your baby a chance to get to know one another and allows you to practice important parenting skills while help is readily available. Mothers who share a room with their baby actually get more rest than mothers who put their baby in a nursery at night.

- **Delay unnecessary tasks**. When your baby's first breastfeeding is delayed, breastfeeding may be more difficult. If possible, avoid all unnecessary tasks such as diapering, bathing, and weighing for at least 1–2 hours after birth.

■ **Choose a comfortable position.** Choose a breastfeeding position
that is comfortable for you and your baby (Figure 14). Turn your
baby on his side or tuck him under your arm so that his chin, chest,
and knees are facing the breast. Using pillows for comfort and support, place your baby at the level of the breast.

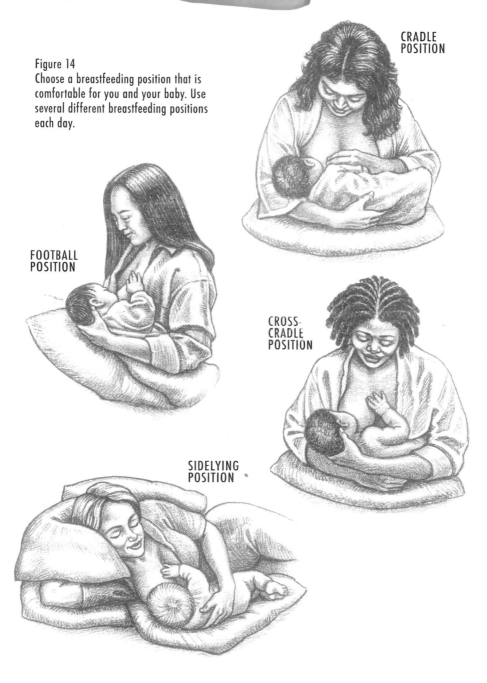

Figure 14
Choose a breastfeeding position that is
comfortable for you and your baby. Use
several different breastfeeding positions
each day.

CRADLE
POSITION

FOOTBALL
POSITION

CROSS-
CRADLE
POSITION

SIDELYING
POSITION

▪ **Support and shape the breast.** If necessary, support and shape the breast with your hand (Figure 15). Place your thumb and fingers opposite one another outside the areola and on the breast. If you gently compress or shape the breast, it may be easier for your baby to latch on. Adjust the position of your thumb and fingers on the breast so that the shaped breast lines up with the widest part of your baby's mouth in the same way that you would position a sandwich in front of your mouth. For example, a mother using the cradle position (baby lying on his side and facing the breast) would shape the breast using a *U-hold* (your hand is shaped like the letter U); while a mother using the football position (baby sitting up and facing the breast) would shape the breast using a *C-hold* (your hand is shaped like the letter C). If you prefer to use the *V-hold,* make sure your thumb and fingers are outside the areola and on the breast (Figure 15).

▪ **Express (gently squeeze out) a few drops of colostrum.** Express a few drops of colostrum before you offer the breast. Your baby will be encouraged to latch on if colostrum is readily available.

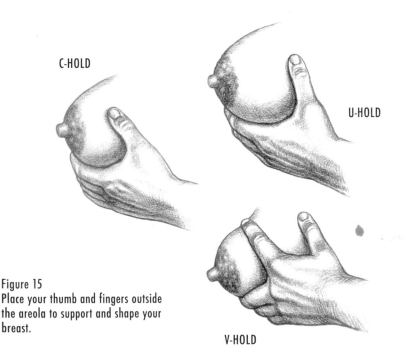

C-HOLD

U-HOLD

Figure 15
Place your thumb and fingers outside the areola to support and shape your breast.

V-HOLD

- **Tickle your baby's nose with your nipple.** To make use of your baby's "rooting reflex," a reflex that causes your baby to open his mouth and seek your breast, gently rub his cheek with your finger or your nipple. Choose the cheek closest to your breast. As your baby turns toward the breast, tickle his nose (or his lips) with your nipple until his mouth opens wide, as if he is yawning.

- **Place your baby on the breast quickly but gently.** Keeping your baby's head and shoulders in a straight line, position his lower lip against your breast and quickly but gently bring him onto the breast. Think about how you position yourself for meals and position your baby the same way—facing the table! If your baby is positioned correctly, he is more likely to get a good, deep latch. Your nipple will point slightly toward the roof of your baby's mouth. Do not lean forward. Bring your baby to you. When your baby is positioned correctly, his tongue should be over his lower gum, between his lower lip and the breast. His lips should curl out, like the lips of a fish, and lie flat against the breast. Hold your baby close to prevent unnecessary pulling on the breast and to keep your baby positioned correctly.

- **Check your areola (darker area around nipple).** When your baby is positioned correctly on the breast, you may see little or none of the areola. How much you see will depend on the size of your areola and the size of your baby's mouth. You may notice that he is slightly off-center on the breast. As a result, you may see more areola on the top, above his lip, and less areola on the bottom.

- **Check your baby's nose, cheeks, and chin.** Your baby's nose and cheeks may gently touch the breast. His chin should press firmly into the breast (Figure 16). Support his shoulders and back with your hand. Place your thumb and fingers below his ears and around his neck. Babies breathe through their nose. If you place your hand on the back of his head, you may press his nose into the breast and make breathing difficult. Women with large breasts can lift up gently on the breast with their fingers below or place a rolled washcloth under the breast to let air enter the nose. Do not press down on the breast with your thumb above, or your nipple may slip out of your baby's mouth.

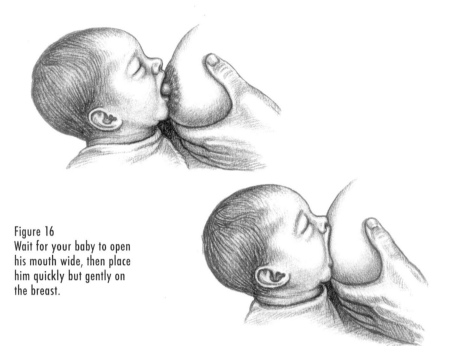

Figure 16
Wait for your baby to open his mouth wide, then place him quickly but gently on the breast.

- **Watch your baby, not the clock.** When your baby stops suckling and swallowing or falls asleep at the first breast, break the suction, burp him, wake him, and offer the second breast.

- **Break the suction.** You can break the suction by gently sliding your finger between your baby's gums and into his mouth. Protect your nipple with your finger as you take your baby off the breast (Figure 17).

- **Burp your baby.** Breastfed babies usually take in less air than bottle-fed babies, so your baby may not burp after every feeding, but it's best to try. You may want to ask your partner to help. Hold your baby upright in your lap or against your shoulder, or place him on his tummy across your lap (Figure 18). Be sure to have a clean cloth handy in case the burp is wet! Gently rub or pat his back. If he hasn't burped after a minute or two, you can offer the second breast.

- **Check your baby's position.** You may feel a tugging sensation when your baby first latches on. However, the tugging sensation should stop after your baby draws your nipple and surrounding breast tissue into his mouth. If the tugging sensation continues, remove your baby from the breast and try again.

Figure 17
Break the suction before
removing your baby from
the breast.

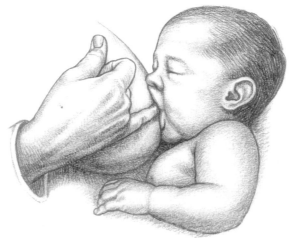

- **Check your nipple**. Your nipple will stretch out (lengthen) when your baby breastfeeds, but the shape of the nipple should look the same before and after he breastfeeds. Some babies are unwilling to latch on well to the tissue around the nipple and latch on to the nipple instead. If your nipple is compressed between the roof of your baby's mouth above and his tongue below, your nipple will look flattened or creased and breastfeeding will be painful!

- **Use a breast pump if needed.** If your nipples are flat or inverted and your baby is unable to maintain a good, deep latch, a breast pump (Figure 12, p. 19) can be used before each breastfeeding to gently pull the nipple out. Choose a hand pump, battery-operated pump, or electric pump, whichever is readily available. Adjust the suction control to the lowest setting, center your nipple in the opening (flange), and apply gentle suction for 10–15 seconds. If necessary, release the suction and repeat the action. As soon as your nipple moves out, remove the pump and quickly put your baby on the breast.

Your Baby's Next Breastfeedings

- **Keep your baby with you day and night.** It may be several hours before your baby wakes to breastfeed again. Many babies breastfeed early and often, but others may show little interest at first. Keep your baby with you day and night while you are in the hospital and during the first 2–4 weeks at home. Look and listen for early signs of hunger or light sleep such as wiggling, lip-smacking, finger-sucking, coughing, or yawning, and offer the breast at those times.

- **Breastfeed 8–12 times in each 24-hour period.** The amount of colostrum taken during early feedings is small (1–3 teaspoons or 5–15 ml), so your baby may seem hungry after feeding and may ask to breastfeed often (every hour). Frequent breastfeeding gives you and your baby a chance to practice this important skill while help is available. Breastfeed 8–12 times in each 24-hour period. Expect to breastfeed every 1–3 hours during the day and every 2–3 hours at night, but remember that every baby is different.

  Some babies will breastfeed every 2–3 hours, day and night, while others will *cluster-feed*, breastfeeding every hour for three to five

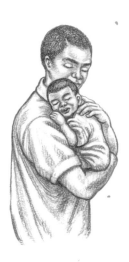
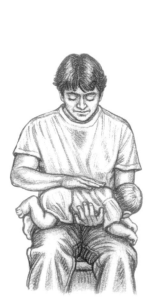
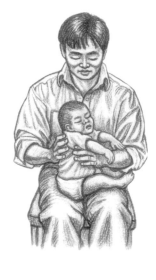

Figure 18
Try different positions
for burping to see what
works best.

feedings and sleeping 3–4 hours between clusters. Some babies will breastfeed for 10–15 minutes on each breast, some will breastfeed for 15–30 minutes on each breast, and others will breastfeed for 15–30 minutes on one breast only. Supplements are seldom necessary unless your baby loses more than 7 percent of his birth weight. Small, frequent feedings make it easier for your baby to adjust to life outside your body.

Breastfed babies are less likely to develop high levels of bilirubin if they breastfeed frequently. Frequent breastfeeding leads to frequent bowel movements, resulting in lower levels of bilirubin and less risk for jaundice.

■ **Wake a sleepy baby.** Sometimes a sleepy baby will not ask to eat often enough. Place him skin-to-skin between your breasts. Watch for early signs of hunger or light sleep and offer the breast at those times. Additional suggestions for waking a sleepy baby include:

- dimming the lights
- unwrapping him
- changing his diaper
- washing his bottom with a cool washcloth
- massaging his feet (my favorite!)
- placing him in your lap in a sitting position, supporting his chin in one hand and massaging his back with the other hand

■ **Relieve fullness and prevent engorgement.** Your milk supply will increase significantly 3–5 days after birth. Your breasts may feel firm and full. Frequent breastfeeding will relieve fullness and prevent engorgement. Breastfeed 8–12 times in each 24-hour period, or every 1–3 hours. Offer both breasts at every feeding, but do not be concerned if your baby seems satisfied with one breast. If necessary, hand express or pump to soften your breasts and relieve the fullness.

■ **Continue to position your baby correctly on the breast.** You might feel soreness when your baby first latches on. However, the soreness should stop as he draws your nipple and the surrounding breast tissue into his mouth. If the soreness continues, remove your baby from the breast and try again.

Remember that when your baby is positioned correctly, his head and chest should be facing the breast. His mouth should be opened wide. His tongue should be over his lower gum, between his lower lip and the breast. His lips should curl out, like the lips of a fish, and lie flat against the breast. His nose and cheeks may gently touch the breast. His chin should press firmly into the breast (Figure 16, p. 26). You may see little or none of the areola. The amount you see will depend on the size of your areola and the size of your baby's mouth.

■ **Know the signs of poor latch.** To transfer milk, your baby must latch on to the breast correctly. When your baby is positioned correctly, your nipple and the surrounding breast tissue should fill your baby's mouth. Your nipple should be at the back of his mouth, with little or no pressure on the nipple itself (Figure 7, p. 12). Your nipple should look the same before and after you breastfeed. When your baby is positioned incorrectly on the breast, nipple pain and damage can occur. Signs of poor latch include:

  • nipples that are flattened or creased after breastfeeding

  • clicking sounds by your baby while breastfeeding

  • dimpling of your baby's cheeks while breastfeeding

  • pain while breastfeeding or between feedings

■ **Know the signs of milk transfer.** When your baby is positioned correctly, your milk ducts (located beneath your areola) are drawn into your baby's mouth and compressed between the roof of his mouth above and his tongue below, forming a sandwich. A wave-like movement of your baby's tongue puts pressure on your milk ducts, causing milk to flow out of the openings in your nipple (Figure 7, p. 12).

The sudden release of milk from the breasts is called the let-down reflex or milk-ejection reflex. Most mothers have more than one let-down per feeding. You may feel a tingling or fullness in the breasts when your milk lets down, or you may notice milk leaking from one breast while your baby breastfeeds from the opposite breast. Don't be concerned if you see or feel nothing; every mother is different. Simply watch your baby. Look and listen for signs of swallowing. When your milk lets down, your baby's sucking pattern will change from short, rapid sucks to a slower, rhythmic, suckle-swallow pattern.

- **Watch your baby, not the clock (Figure 19).** Breastfeed as long as your baby wishes on the first breast before you offer the second breast. This is called *baby-led feeding*. If you limit the length of breast-feedings, your baby may not get enough high-fat milk. When your baby stops suckling and swallowing or falls asleep at the first breast, break the suction, burp him, wake him, and offer the second breast.

- **Break the suction.** Break the suction by gently sliding your finger between your baby's gums to the tip of your nipple (Figure 17). Protect your nipple with your finger as you take your baby off the breast.

- **Offer both breasts at each feeding.** Offer both breasts at each feeding, but do not be concerned if your baby seems satisfied with one breast. Each breast can provide a full meal. If necessary, hand express or pump to relieve the fullness in the second breast. If your baby breastfeeds poorly on the first breast and shows no sign of suckling and swallowing, offer the first breast again. To increase the flow of milk, gently compress the breast between your thumb and fingers when your baby pauses from feeding. Breastfeed well on one breast before you offer the second breast.

- **Begin each feeding on the breast offered last.**

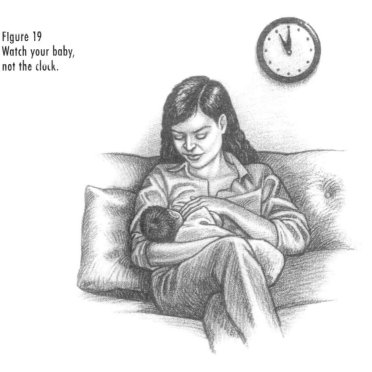

Figure 19
Watch your baby,
not the clock.

■ **Use breastfeeding positions that work best for you and your baby.**
Support your baby well in whatever positions you choose (Figure 14,
p. 23). This will prevent unnecessary pulling on the breast, keep
your baby positioned correctly, and prevent nipple soreness.

■ **Avoid artificial nipples.** Wait until you and your baby have learned
to breastfeed well (4–6 weeks) before offering a bottle or pacifier.
Bottle nipples and pacifiers may confuse your baby.

■ **Avoid water or formula supplements.** Your breastmilk is all your baby
needs for the first 6 months. Frequent use of water or formula supplements can decrease your milk supply and lead to early *weaning* (stopping breastfeeding). If giving a supplement is necessary for medical
reasons, choose a method that is least likely to interfere with your
baby's ability to breastfeed later. For example, you can supplement at
the breast with a supplemental feeding device or feeding tube and
syringe, or you can supplement away from the breast using a spoon,
eye dropper, or cup. If you decide to use an artificial nipple, choose a
nipple that is soft and supple with a wide base and a slow flow.

■ **Keep a daily log.** During the first 2–4 weeks, while you and your
baby are learning to breastfeed, you may want to keep a daily log of
your baby's wet diapers, bowel movements (poops), and breastfeedings (Figure 20). Knowing what to expect during the early weeks
will give you confidence in your ability to breastfeed and let you
know when to seek help.

• Expect 8 to 12 breastfeedings in each 24 hours.

• Expect clear or pale yellow urine and six or more wet diapers a
day by day 5.

• After day 1, expect at least three stools a day for the next 3 days
and at least four stools a day for the following 4 weeks.

• Your baby's stools will be black and sticky (*meconium*) on days 1 and
2, green and pasty on days 3 and 4, and yellow, seedy, and runny
by day 5.

• Breastfed babies' stools look like a mixture of water, yellow
mustard, cottage cheese, and sesame seeds!

• Expect small, frequent, runny stools with very little solid material.
Sometimes, all you see is a yellow stain in the diaper the size of
your baby's fist.

- After the first 4–6 weeks, expect larger and fewer stools. Many babies have one large stool every 1–5 days, though others continue to have small, frequent stools each day for many months.

■ **Keep track of your baby's weight.** Your baby's health care provider will weigh your baby during each health check.

- Expect your baby to lose no more than 7 percent of his birth weight during the first 5 days.

- Expect your baby to be back to his birth weight by 10 days of age.

- After the first week, expect your baby to gain 4–8 ounces each week during the first 3 months.

Figure 20
Daily log.

Day	8-12 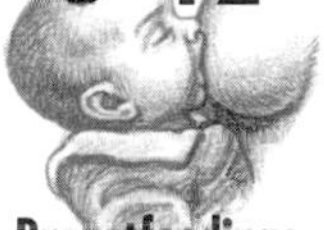 Breastfeedings	6-8 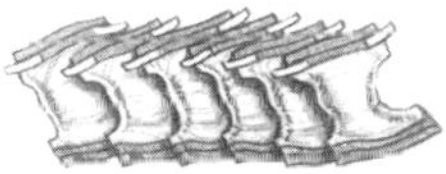 Wet Diapers	3-4 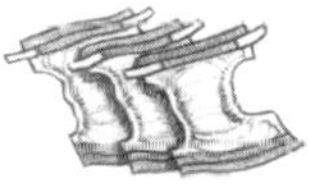 Poops
(Sample)	ʮ ʮ I	ʮ I	IIII
Mon.			
Tues.			
Wed.			
Thurs.			
Fri.			
Sat.			
Sun.			

5

Continuing to Breastfeed

Congratulations! You Made It!

In the first weeks after birth, focus on taking care of yourself and your baby. Leave household chores to others—cobblers and cobwebs can wait! Nap at least once a day when your baby naps, and wear your pajamas or nightgown during the first week as a reminder to family and friends that you are still recovering from pregnancy, labor, and birth. Accept all offers of help, and don't hesitate to *ask* for help. The frustrations of parenting seem greater when parents are worn out from too little sleep.

If necessary, limit visitors and the length of visits. Place a small "Do Not Disturb" sign on the front door to discourage unwanted guests.

Though some mothers are comfortable breastfeeding in front of family and friends (both male and female), many are not. It is important that you be relaxed. So don't hesitate to speak up if you need more privacy.

Though it is nice to have help at home, family and friends can be a source of stress if their knowledge of breastfeeding is limited. You may need to explain politely the benefits of breastfeeding and the importance of frequent feedings, feeding on request, and nighttime feedings. Explain that it is better for you and your baby to nap during the day and breastfeed at night than for Grandma to bottle-feed your baby so that you can sleep through the night.

Eat a variety of healthy foods, and drink to satisfy your thirst. If your urine is clear or pale yellow in color, you will know that you are drinking enough fluid. Use each breastfeeding as a reminder to eat a light snack or drink a beverage. You can begin light exercise 2–4 weeks after birth. However, listen to what your body tells you. Many mothers, eager to resume their active lifestyles, do too much too soon and quickly regret it. Remember, these early weeks are a learning experience for the whole family, so relax and enjoy this time together.

Getting to Know Your Breastfed Baby

The First 6 Months

Every baby has basic needs—food, oxygen, warmth, safety, and love. You will know your baby's needs are met if you understand how normal breastfed babies behave. If you have family members or friends who have breastfed, watching them with their babies may have taught you a lot about newborn behavior. But if most mothers you know have not breastfed, or have breastfed for only a short time, you may have much to learn.

During the first 3 months, your baby grows very fast, so he needs lots of calories. Since your baby's stomach is the size of his fist, it is easy to understand why he needs to eat often (every 1–3 hours). Watch your baby for early signs of hunger and offer the breast at those times. If you offer your breast while your baby is quiet but alert, he is more likely to latch on and breastfeed well. Crying is the last sign of hunger and should be avoided. If your baby has to cry to be fed, you will often find that he breastfeeds poorly and falls asleep at the breast after only a minute or two. You can be sure that your baby is getting enough to eat if he has small, frequent poops (three to four each day), heavy, wet diapers (six to eight each day), and steady weight gain (4–8 ounces each week).

Once your baby is breastfeeding well and gaining weight, you can begin to let him set his own feeding schedule. This may happen at about 4–6 weeks after birth. But remember that every baby is different. Some babies will continue to breastfeed every 2–3 hours day and night for many weeks. Other babies will breastfeed every 1–2 hours when awake and sleep for longer periods of time.

If your baby sleeps for 4 hours or more at a time during the early weeks, you may need to express enough milk to relieve fullness, prevent engorgement, and maintain your milk supply. Expressed breastmilk can be stored in the refrigerator or freezer for later use. As your baby's feeding pattern changes, your breasts will respond to your baby's changing needs and make just the right amount of milk. Breasts truly are amazing!

Many parents want to know when their babies will sleep through the night. It is important to remember that every baby is different. When your baby is 6–12 weeks old, he will usually sleep for 4–5 hours at night. You can try to calm your baby and lengthen the period of time between feedings at night by diapering, walking, and rocking. Many babies sleep for 6 hours at night starting around 6 months of age. Your definition of "night" may need to change! As your baby gets older, he will sleep for a longer period of time at night.

You may wonder if you can sleep with your baby. Research shows that when babies and mothers sleep near one another, nighttime feedings are easier, mothers get more sleep, and babies have less risk of sudden infant death syndrome (SIDS), the sudden, unexplained death of an infant between 1 month and 1 year of age. Babies often sleep in more than one place, including car seats, cribs, cots, bassinets, co-sleepers (baby beds that attach to the side of adult beds), and adult beds. While some sleep areas are safe, others are not. Certain conditions and behaviors can make a safe area an unsafe one. The following suggestions will help you and your baby sleep safely.

- Do not sleep with your baby on sofas or overstuffed chairs.

- Do not place your baby alone in an adult bed.

- Do not place your baby in an adult bed with older siblings.

- Parents who smoke should not sleep with their baby. Cigarette smoke increases the risk of SIDS.

- Parents who have used alcohol or drugs should not sleep with their baby.

- Parents who are extremely overweight should not sleep with their baby.

When mothers and babies sleep near one another, babies breastfeed more often and have fewer periods of deep sleep. Less deep sleep may decrease the risk of SIDS. To further decrease the risk of SIDS, follow the suggestions below.

- Place your baby on his back to sleep. Do not place your baby on his tummy or on his side. If your baby has a medical condition that prevents him from sleeping on his back, talk with your baby's doctor about a safe sleeping position.

- Place your baby on a firm mattress or other firm surface to sleep.

- Use *only* a lightweight cover or blanket in your baby's bed, or place your baby in a sleep sack. Do not use a comforter, duvet, quilt, or pillow.

- Keep your baby comfortable. Do not let your baby get too hot. Use a single layer of clothing in addition to his diaper.

- Keep your baby in a smoke-free place for at least the first year of his life.

- Take your baby for regular health checks and immunizations.

- Call your baby's doctor right away if your baby seems sick.

After 6 Months

Breastmilk is the only food your baby needs for the first 6 months of life. During the second half of the first year, breastmilk remains an important part of your baby's diet, along with iron-rich solid foods. If breastmilk is not provided throughout the first year, iron fortified infant formula is recommended. Cow's milk should not be used until your baby is at least 1 year old.

Breastfeeding provides benefits beyond the first year and should continue as long as mother, father, and baby wish. Breastfeeding beyond the first year is common in many parts of the world. In the United States, where breasts are seen mainly as sexual objects, women who breastfeed in public or beyond the first year sometimes get dirty looks or hear nasty comments. In some states there are laws that protect a woman's right to breastfeed in public.

If you are shy or easily embarrassed, choose a private place where you will not be disturbed, and wear clothing that makes it possible to breastfeed without being noticed. If you choose to breastfeed in public, it may encourage other mothers to do the same. In the meantime, be confident in knowing that you are giving your baby the very best—nutritionally, immunologically, and emotionally.

6 Eating for Two

Mothers have many questions concerning nutrition during breastfeeding.

"How many calories should I eat while breastfeeding?"

"How can I lose the extra weight I gained during my pregnancy?"

"Are vitamin and mineral supplements necessary?"

Though some health care providers recommend a strict diet for breast-feeding mothers, others suggest that mothers eat whatever they want. The following questions and answers may help you decide which foods are best for you and your baby.

Do I need to eat more calories while I am breastfeeding?

Nutritional needs depend on how much milk is produced. For example, the woman who gives her baby formula in addition to breastmilk does not need as many calories as the woman who breastfeeds twins. Milk production requires about 500–1,000 calories per day. Half the calories come from body fat stored during pregnancy, the other half come from foods that you eat. Some nutritionists recommend that women eat 500 additional calories each day while breastfeeding. However, most women can produce enough milk while eating about the same number of calories as they did before they were pregnant. If you want to lose the weight that you gained during pregnancy, you should avoid high-calorie foods with no nutritional value.

Eat to satisfy your hunger and try not to lose weight until your milk supply is well established—about 4–6 weeks after birth. It is important to remember that the more you breastfeed, the more calories your body uses. The best weight loss is achieved when you breastfeed exclusively or almost exclusively for 6 months.

How can I lose the extra weight I gained during my pregnancy?

Most women find that over a 6-month period they lose the extra weight gained during pregnancy. Though this may seem like a long time, restricting calories to lose weight more quickly is not recommended since it can interfere with milk production. Although even malnourished mothers can produce high-quality milk, production is often at the expense of a mother's own health. By eating enough calories, you help ensure that your need for other nutrients, such as protein, vitamins, and minerals, is met as well.

If you were overweight before your pregnancy, breastfeeding can help you lose weight. Once your milk supply is stable, eating 1,800 calories a day will maintain your milk supply and allow you to lose weight. If you do aerobic exercise or are very tall, you may need 2,000–2,400 calories a day. The best guide to use is how fast you lose weight. Women who are very overweight should not lose more than 4–6 pounds a month. Women who need to lose 25 pounds or less should not lose more than 3–4 pounds a month.

If you were the right weight-for-height before your pregnancy, you will find that eating to satisfy your hunger and breastfeeding exclusively for 6 months will result in a gradual return to your pre-pregnancy weight. As your baby reaches 6 months of age, you may find that you need to add calories to your diet to keep from losing too much weight. Remember that the minimum number of calories recommended is 1,800 each day. Again, women who are physically active or very tall may need 2,000–2,400 calories.

If you were underweight before your pregnancy, you may need to add calories above your usual intake in order to keep from losing too much weight. This is especially important as your baby gets older, if you are exclusively breastfeeding. Weighing less than you did before your pregnancy should be avoided.

need to drink extra fluid while I am breastfeeding?

Your thirst is the best signal of how much fluid you should drink. In fact, excess fluids can actually decrease milk production. So follow your own thirst (about six to eight servings of fluids a day) and drink healthy beverages such as water, low-fat or nonfat milk, and 100 percent fruit or vegetable juice. You can be sure you are getting enough to drink if your urine is clear or pale yellow.

Do I need to take vitamin and mineral supplements while I am breastfeeding?

As long as you eat a balanced diet that includes a variety of foods, the only supplement you may need to take while breastfeeding is iron. Even if you do not menstruate (bleed each month) while exclusively breastfeeding, extra iron helps to replace the iron used during pregnancy.

If you have iron deficiency or iron deficiency anemia, your doctor will prescribe an iron supplement (60–120 mg a day). Remember that iron supplements are best absorbed on an empty stomach and should not be taken at the same time you take other nutrient supplements.

Some women avoid dairy products because of lactose intolerance, milk protein allergy, dislike of dairy products, or vegan diet (strict vegetarian diet that does not include milk products). *If you do not eat dairy products or other high-calcium foods each day,* you should take a calcium supplement (600 mg a day).

Fortified dairy products are a source of vitamin D. *If you avoid dairy products and get less than 30 minutes of sun exposure a week,* you should take a vitamin D supplement (5–10 mg or 200–400 IU). The ultraviolet rays of the sun (with some help from the liver and kidneys) change a substance in the skin into vitamin D. Sunscreen blocks ultraviolet rays, so if you depend on sunlight for your vitamin D, wait for 30 minutes outdoors before you apply sunscreen. If you are in the sun often, you can wait less than 30 minutes.

Women who do not eat animal protein (meat, fish, eggs, or milk products) must choose foods carefully to get enough calories, protein, and nutrients, especially vitamin B_{12}, iron, vitamin D, and zinc. Protein and nutrients can be obtained by eating soy products and a variety of seeds, nuts, grains, legumes, vegetables, and cereals.

Do I need to limit the amount of fat in my diet?

You can limit the amount of fat in your diet by eating reduced-fat and nonfat foods such as mayonnaise, cream cheese, salad dressings, and cheese. But be sure to get some fat in your diet. If you are eating the minimum number of calories (1,800 a day), your diet should include 60 grams of fat. This may seem like a lot, but it is not. Every animal product you eat except for nonfat dairy products has fat. Lean chicken provides 2–3 grams of fat per ounce of meat. Beef and pork have 5–8 grams of fat per ounce. Fish has 1–5 grams of fat. Depending on the choices you make, it is easy to get 6–48 grams of fat from two small servings (3 ounces each) of high-protein foods per day. Balance a higher-fat protein choice with a lower-fat protein choice at the next meal.

You can limit the amount of saturated fat (the type in animal products) in your diet by keeping your protein servings small (2–4 ounces) and using monounsaturated and polyunsaturated oils in cooking. These *good* oils include olive, canola, sesame, corn, soybean, safflower, and walnut. Remember, oils have 5 grams of fat per teaspoon. Also, read labels on products such as mayonnaise, margarine, sour cream, and processed foods to check their fat content.

How can I increase the fatty acid content of my milk?

While the total amount of fat and the types of fatty acids in human milk may vary from one mother to another, human milk contains all the fatty acids a healthy, full-term baby needs. Some fatty acids cannot be made in the body and must be obtained from food sources. These are the *essential* fatty acids. Others, like the long-chain polyunsaturated fatty acids, are made in the body but are also available in foods. Two long-chain polyunsaturated fatty acids that play an important role in visual development and brain function are docosahexaenoic acid (DHA) and arachidonic acid (ARA). To ensure that your milk contains adequate amounts of DHA and ARA, include fatty fish (salmon, canned tuna, sardines, herring, anchovies) and vegetable oils (olive, canola, corn, safflower) in your diet.

Do I need to limit the amount of fish in my diet?

Fish are a good source of high-quality protein and are low in saturated fat. But nearly all fish contain mercury. So think small! Large fish that feed on smaller fish (swordfish, king mackerel, tilefish, shark, and tuna) often have high levels of mercury and should be eaten no more than once a month.

Farm-raised fish (especially salmon) are usually fed ground-up fish that contain high levels of PCBs and other cancer-causing chemicals. Many producers of farm-raised fish are trying improve the quality of the food that is fed to their fish. Because few fish are labeled, it is hard to tell if fish are farm-raised or caught in the wild. Farm-raised fish should be eaten no more than once or twice a month.

You can still enjoy the health benefits of seafood by eating shellfish (shrimp, scallops, crab, squid, and lobster), canned fish (sardines, herring, and anchovies), or smaller ocean fish (wild salmon, cod, and sole).

Is it true that some foods can make my baby fussy?

Occasionally something in your diet may make your baby fussy. Foods that sometimes cause fussiness include milk products, eggs, and nuts. If you have a family history of allergic disease or a very fussy baby, you might want to limit these foods in your diet.

Small amounts of caffeine (the equivalent of one or two cups of regular coffee a day) are considered safe for breastfeeding mothers and healthy, full-term babies. But large amounts of caffeine (the equivalent of five or more cups of regular coffee a day) can cause fussy, wakeful babies. If you have a fussy baby, you might want to limit your intake of caffeine-containing drinks and foods such as coffee, tea, chocolate, and some carbonated beverages (see Table 1). The amount of caffeine in a cup of coffee or tea depends upon the equipment used for brewing and the ingredients.

Can I use artificial sweeteners while I am breastfeeding?

Small amounts of artificial sweeteners such as saccharin and aspartame are thought to be safe. Saccharin is a weak cancer-causing substance.

Table 1. Caffeine Content of Drinks and Foods

DRINK/FOOD	CAFFEINE
Brewed drip coffee / 7 ounces	115–175 mg
Brewed percolator coffee / 7 ounces	80–135 mg
Instant coffee / 7 ounces	65–100 mg
Brewed tea / 7 ounces	40–60 mg
Instant tea / 7 ounces	30 mg
Iced tea / 12 ounces	70 mg
Mountain Dew / 12 ounces	54 mg
Mello Yello / 12 ounces	53 mg
Coca-Cola / 12 ounces	46 mg
Diet Coke / 12 ounces	46 mg
Dr. Pepper / 12 ounces	40 mg
Pepsi-Cola / 12 ounces	30 mg
Diet Pepsi / 12 ounces	36 mg
Milk chocolate / 1 ounce	6 mg
Dark chocolate / 1 ounce	20 mg

The safe level of daily intake is 500 mg for children and 1,000 mg for adults. A popular brand of artificial sweetener using saccharin has about 14–20 mg per packet.

Aspartame causes an increase in the level of phenylalanine and should not be used by individuals with phenylketonuria (PKU). There is no proof that aspartame harms breastfed babies, but moderate use (no more than two to four servings a day) of artificial sweeteners and artificially sweetened beverages is recommended.

Can I drink alcohol while breastfeeding?

Drinking small amounts of alcohol (8 ounces of wine, 24 ounces of beer, or 2 1/2 ounces of spirits such as whiskey, rum, vodka, or gin) no more than once a week is thought to be safe. However, alcohol can change the flavor of your milk, shorten your breastfeeding sessions, decrease your milk supply, and limit your baby's weight gain. Daily use of alcohol, even in small amounts, can affect your baby's motor development and your ability to care for your baby. To limit the effects of alcohol on you and your baby, drink no more than one or two drinks a week and try not to breastfeed for at least 2 hours after you drink.

Can I smoke while I am breastfeeding?

Smoking affects the breastfeeding mother and baby in many ways. It lowers the nutritional status of the mother, decreases the metabolism of vitamin B_{12}, alters zinc balance in the body, and lowers the levels of vitamin C and folic acid. Smoking causes a decrease in prolactin and oxytocin, a decrease in the fat content of milk, and a decrease in milk production, which can lead to early weaning. Because the benefits of breastfeeding outweigh the risks of smoking, mothers who smoke are still encouraged to breastfeed. However, to limit the effects of second-hand smoke on your baby, reduce the number of cigarettes you smoke to no more than five a day, and do not smoke in the house, in the car, or near your baby.

How can I improve my diet to produce the highest quality milk possible?

- Eat the recommended number of servings (see Table 2).

- Eat a fish meal (especially cold water fish like salmon) two or three times a week. If you eat fish that contain high levels of mercury (like swordfish) limit your intake to no more than once a month.

- Use nonfat milk products and a variety of oils.

- Eat a minimum of 1,800 calories a day.

- Select foods that provide important nutrients (see Table 3).

Table 2. Suggested Breastfeeding Diet

FOOD GROUP	NUMBER OF SERVINGS	EXAMPLES OF ONE SERVING
BREAD, CEREAL, RICE, PASTA Whole-grain products are best	6–11	1 slice bread $1/2$ roll, muffin, biscuit 1 tortilla $1/2$ cup hot cereal 1 cup ready-to-eat cereal $1/2$ cup rice, noodles, pasta
FRUITS High-fiber fruits are best	2–4	$3/4$ cup fruit juice 1 medium orange, apple, banana, pear $1/2$ grapefruit $1/2$ cup chopped, cooked, or canned fruit $1/2$ cup berries 1 slice melon $1/4$ cup dried fruit
VEGETABLES High fiber vegetables are best	3–5	$3/4$ cup vegetable juice $1/2$ cup cooked vegetables such as broccoli, green beans, peas, turnip greens, kale $1/2$ cup chopped raw vegetables 1 cup raw leafy vegetables such as spinach, lettuce, endive
MEAT, POULTRY, FISH, DRY BEANS/ PEAS, EGGS, NUTS	3	2–3 ounces lean meat, fish, poultry 1 egg $1/2$ cup cooked beans 2 tablespoons peanut butter $1/2$ cup canned tuna $1/2$ cup tofu $2 1/2$ ounces soy burger $1/3$ cup nuts or seeds
MILK/MILK PRODUCTS	3–4	1 cup milk 1 cup yogurt $1 1/2$ cups cottage cheese $1 1/2$ ounces natural cheese 2 ounces processed cheese such as American $1 1/2$ cups ice cream
FATS, OILS	Small amounts	1 teaspoon butter, mayonnaise, oil 1 tablespoon salad dressing 1 tablespoon sour cream

Table 3. Foods Containing Important Nutrients

FOLIC ACID	CALCIUM	VITAMIN C
leafy vegetables	milk	citrus fruits and juices
green beans	yogurt	fortified juices
legumes	cheese	strawberries
fortified cereals	sardines/salmon with bones	broccoli
fruit	dark green leafy vegetables	cabbage
	dried beans and peas	potatoes
	fortified orange juice	green peppers
	fortified tofu	
	fortified tortillas	

ZINC	VITAMIN A	VITAMIN B
beef	dark green leafy vegetables	banana
poultry	orange/yellow vegetables	watermelon
seafood	liver	meat
eggs	egg yolk	potatoes
pork	cheese	sweet potatoes
fortified cereals	milk	nuts/seeds
yogurt	butter	fortified cereals
legumes		
seeds		

7

Especially for Fathers

Becoming a Family

Families come in all shapes and sizes—grandparents, fathers, mothers, brothers, sisters, boyfriends, girlfriends, and best friends. You can have a family of two, three, four, or more. No matter what type of family you have, the arrival of a new baby triggers a wide range of emotions. Becoming a family takes time and patience. Try to relax and enjoy each moment because it doesn't get any easier than this!

Breastfeeding benefits everyone who is an important part of your baby's life. A breastfed baby, warm and snug against your chest, gives you confidence in your ability to calm your baby. Nighttime feedings are simple when there is no formula to mix, measure, or warm. In addition, breastfed babies are portable, good news for families on the go.

Learning to Breastfeed

While making milk is natural, breastfeeding is a skill that must be learned. Sometimes a mother and baby know just what to do, but more often they need to be taught. By learning all that you can during pregnancy, you will be better able to help after your baby is born. This book will answer most of your questions, so be sure to read it carefully and keep it handy.

Encourage your partner to practice breastfeeding as often as she can while she is in the hospital. Plan to spend the night at the hospital with her if there is enough room. Keep your baby with you as much as possible and ask every question that comes to mind. Watch as the nurses and lactation consultants help your partner with breastfeeding, and ask them to show you how you can help.

Remember that mothers and babies need to breastfeed frequently and rest often, so you may need to limit the number of visitors and the length of visits. Take advantage of this time together to get to know one another. There will be plenty of time later for family and friends.

Accepting Help with Household Chores

Accept all offers of help from persons willing to cook, clean, do laundry, shop for food, or care for your partner. Refuse all offers of help from persons who are interested only in caring for your baby. If you are going to become confident in your ability to care for your baby, you and your partner need to practice your parenting skills. Grandma already knows how to care for babies; now it is time for you and your partner to learn. But be sure to tell Grandma how much you appreciate her help as you learn to be a parent to her grandchild.

Getting to Know Your Baby!

Breastfeeding is an important part of parenting, but equally important is the time you spend with your baby and the special moments you share (Figure 21). Find something that you enjoy doing with your baby and make it a routine. Taking walks, splashing in the tub, listening to music, playing games, or simply watching TV or reading the newspaper are ways for you and your baby to spend time together and to get to know one another.

Returning to "Normal"

Many parents ask, "When will things get back to *normal?*" The truth is, never! Your idea of normal will need to change. You will need to adjust priorities and establish goals for a life that now includes another person. There may be little time at first for individual needs. However, as you learn to be a parent to your baby, remember to be a friend and lover to your partner.

Despite all your efforts there will be times when things do not go well. Be prepared for the day when you arrive home to find your partner still in her nightgown. She and the baby are crying, the laundry needs to

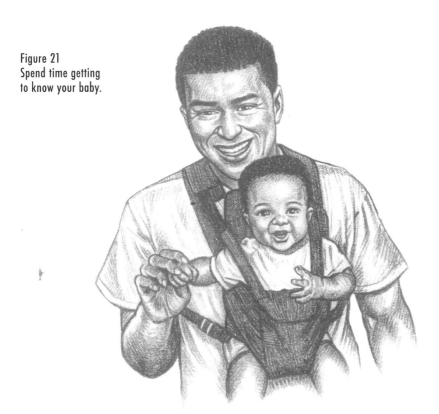

Figure 21
Spend time getting
to know your baby.

be done, and there is no dinner. Perhaps your day was just as bad! Instead of getting angry, put a load of clothes in the washing machine, take the baby for a walk (it will relax all of you), order food for dinner, and suggest that your partner make a cup of tea and take a warm bath. She will love you for understanding, and it will keep you both from saying things you might later regret.

Providing Encouragement and Support

In Chapter 1, "Benefits of Breastfeeding," you learned that breastfeeding is good for babies, mothers, and fathers. (If you haven't read Chapter 1 yet, it's not too late!) Mothers are 10 times more likely to breastfeed if they have the support of their partner.

So why doesn't every father encourage his partner to breastfeed? The fact is that most fathers do support breastfeeding—at first. But early support for breastfeeding is often short-lived. If you know how other fathers feel, you may be better able to manage your feelings. Some comments from fathers appear below.

"I feel so helpless. I can't even calm the baby."

"I didn't realize how much I would miss the quiet nights and childless days."

"Sometimes I'm angry at the baby for changing our lives."

"Sometimes I'm angry at my partner for spending so much time with the baby."

Perhaps you were secretly hoping that your partner would choose to bottle-feed or would breastfeed for only a short time.

Perhaps you are shy or easily embarrassed and feel uncomfortable when your partner breastfeeds in front of family and friends.

Perhaps you are concerned that breastfeeding is taking too much time.

The truth is that parenting takes time and energy no matter how you choose to feed your baby.

Managing Negative Feelings

So how do you manage negative feelings if they occur? You can begin by realizing that fathers play a greater role than anyone else in not just a mother's decision to breastfeed but also in her choice to continue breastfeeding. When a group of mothers were asked to name the *one* factor that most influenced their choice to breastfeed, 9 out of 10 mothers identified the feeding preference of their partner. That makes you a VIP (very important person) whether you realize it or not! If you are comfortable talking with other fathers about your feelings, you may be surprised to learn that they have many of the same feelings. Parenting is a learning experience for mothers, fathers, and babies.

Even though breastfeeding may take more time than you had expected, it is still the best choice for your partner, your baby, and you. For those fathers eager to feed their babies, it may help to remember that the period of exclusive breastfeeding is only 6 months (less than a football season!) and that when the time is right, fathers can be the first to offer solid foods. Even before 6 months, you can offer expressed (pumped) breastmilk in a cup or bottle, depending on your baby's age and ability. If you offer a cup or bottle too soon, you can confuse your baby, so wait until your baby is breastfeeding well (at least 4–6 weeks after birth).

Parenting is never easy, so relax and enjoy this time together. Parenting a breastfed baby is a special joy, the benefits of which last a lifetime.

Remembering What You Have Learned

The following list summarizes all the ways in which you can help to make breastfeeding the right choice for you and your partner.

- Learn as much as you can during pregnancy about the benefits of breastfeeding and the risks of not breastfeeding.

- Attend prenatal breastfeeding classes, childbirth classes, and parenting classes.

- Talk with other fathers about their breastfeeding experiences. Share your thoughts and feelings and encourage them to share theirs.

- Plan prenatal visits so that you can be present. Listen to what the doctor says and ask questions. Get to know your baby before he is born.

- After your baby is born, watch how others help with breastfeeding and ask them to show you.

- Limit visitors and the length of visits.

- Watch your baby for early signs of hunger (sucking sounds, hand-to-mouth movements, wiggling, squirming) and bring your baby to your partner to breastfeed.

- Help your partner position your baby at the breast. Use extra pillows for support. Be sure that your partner is comfortable and relaxed.

- Bring your partner water or juice and a healthy snack to eat while she breastfeeds.

■ Keep your partner company during breastfeedings. Let her know that you would like to burp and diaper the baby.

■ Tell your partner what a wonderful mother she is and what a great job she is doing.

■ Ask your partner to make a list of household chores that need to be done. Decide which chores you can do and ask family and friends to help with others.

■ Make dinner. Or you can dine on takeout!

■ Take the baby for a period of time each day so that your partner can nap, bathe, read, or simply relax. Use this time to get to know your baby.

■ Plan time alone with your partner. Ask someone you trust to care for your baby. Let your partner know that she is still an important part of your life.

■ Talk with your partner about how you feel and about how she feels.

■ Keep your sense of humor—laughter is truly the best medicine!

■ If your partner is returning to work outside the home, go shopping together to buy a breast pump and milk storage containers. Discuss ways that you can make the return to work easier. See Chapter 16, "Combining Breastfeeding and Working," for more suggestions.

Babies change everything. They turn your life inside out and upside down. You will never be the person you were before. You will be a father instead. One day your baby will know how lucky he is to have you for a father. And through your support of breastfeeding, you will know that you have given your baby the best from the very beginning.

8 Managing Possible Problems

The more you learn about how to breastfeed, the less likely you are to have problems while breastfeeding. It is best to prevent problems before they occur. But sometimes, despite your best efforts, problems happen. If you know what signs to look for you can pick up on problems early and start treatment right away.

Breast Engorgement

Signs

Nearly all women experience breast fullness during the first 2–3 days after their babies are born. Do not confuse normal fullness with engorgement. Engorged breasts are swollen, hard, and painful, and your skin is red, shiny, and hot. Your body temperature can increase slightly (to less than 100° F or 37.7° C).

Cause

After your baby is born, your blood carries fluid and nutrients to the breasts so that you can make enough milk to meet your baby's needs. This added fluid causes the breasts to swell. Frequent breastfeedings or milk expression will reduce the swelling and soften the breasts. If breastfeedings are infrequent, delayed, or missed, the breasts overfill and fluid collects in the breast tissue, causing engorgement.

Recommended Treatment

- Put cold packs on your breasts to reduce the swelling. Bags of frozen peas wrapped in a wet washcloth work well. Some women

use cold, raw cabbage leaves on the breasts after each feeding to
reduce engorgement. Why cabbage leaves relieve engorgement is
unclear. There may be a substance in the leaves that reduces
swelling, or the cool temperature of the leaves may be the cause.
Rinse the leaves in cold water before use. Place the leaves on the
breasts with the nipples exposed until the leaves wilt. Apply fresh
leaves only until the swelling decreases.

■ Hand express or pump a small amount of colostrum or milk. This
will soften your breasts and make it easier for your baby to latch on
correctly (see "Hand Expressing," p. 141). If your breasts are leaking
freely, taking a warm shower or tub bath or soaking the breasts in a
pan of warm water may make milk expression easier. It is important
to remember that heat can increase swelling, so do not use heat
unless your breasts are leaking freely.

■ Breastfeed every 1–3 hours during the day and every 2–3 hours at
night. To increase the flow of milk, gently massage the breast in a
circular pattern while your baby is breastfeeding, using the flat part
of your fingers (Figure 22). If your breasts are still full and firm after
feeding, hand express or pump to relieve fullness.

Figure 22
Massage your breast to
encourage the flow of milk
and relieve fullness.

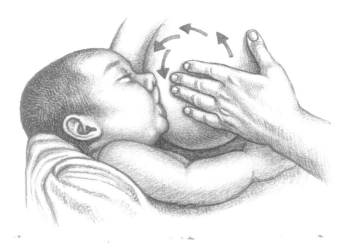

- Wear a bra for comfort and support. Avoid bras that are too tight or that bind, making it difficult to relieve fullness and soften the breasts. Avoid bras with underwires. If you prefer a bra with underwires, remove the bra for one or two feedings during the day and at night.

To Prevent Engorgement

- Breastfeed as soon as possible after birth.

- Breastfeed every 1–3 hours during the day and every 2–3 hours at night. Do not skip nighttime feedings.

- Breastfeed as long as your baby wishes on the first breast before offering the second breast. If necessary, hand express or pump to relieve fullness in the second breast.

- Offer both breasts at every feeding.

- Begin each feeding on the breast offered last.

- If you delay or miss a feeding or your baby breastfeeds poorly, hand express or pump to relieve fullness.

- Avoid the use of water or formula supplements.

Sore Nipples

Signs

Breast or nipple soreness can occur during or between breastfeedings. Nipples are pink, red, or purple. You may see a break in the skin at the base of the nipple or on the top of the nipple. Thick, yellow material draining from the damaged area can be a sign of infection.

Cause

Nipple soreness can occur any time, but it is most likely to occur during the first or second week of breastfeeding. Soreness usually occurs at the beginning of a feeding when your baby latches on to the breast and draws the nipple and areola into his mouth. If your baby is positioned well on the breast, the soreness will last only a few seconds. If your baby is positioned incorrectly on the breast, the soreness will continue and nipple damage can occur. Other causes of nipple soreness include breast engorgement, breast infection, the use of creams or ointments, and the misuse of nipple shields or breast pumps.

Recommended Treatment

- Position your baby correctly on the breast (Figure 6, p. 11). Turn your baby on his side or tuck him under your arm so that his face, chest, and knees are facing your breast. Use pillows to support your baby at the level of your breast. Sit back and relax. Bring your baby to you. Tickle his nose (or his lips) with your nipple until his mouth opens wide. Position your baby's lower lip against your breast and quickly but gently place your baby on the breast. Don't let him nibble his way on. His tongue should be over his lower gum, between his lower lip and the breast. His lips should turn out, like the lips of a fish, and lie flat against the breast. His chin should press firmly into the breast. His nose and cheeks may gently touch the breast.

- If necessary, express a small amount of milk or colostrum to soften the breast before you allow your baby to latch on.

- Begin each feeding on the breast that is the least sore. When a let-down reflex occurs and milk begins to flow, move your baby to the sore breast and breastfeed just long enough to relieve the fullness and soften the breast. If both breasts are sore, use a warm, wet washcloth and gentle massage to start the flow of milk before you offer your baby the breast.

- If necessary, limit the length of each breastfeeding on the sore breast and breastfeed more often, every 1–2 hours. Hand express to relieve fullness.

- Hold your baby close to prevent unnecessary pulling on the breast. Remember to break the suction before removing your baby from the breast.

- After each breastfeeding, put a small amount of colostrum or breast-milk on the areola and nipple of each breast (Figure 23).

- Wash your breasts and nipples once a day with a mild antibacterial soap and water. Do not wash your nipples before each breastfeeding. Even water, used often, will dry the skin.

- Avoid using creams, lotions, and oils. If your nipples crack or bleed, check with your doctor, lactation consultant, or nurse before putting anything on the damaged nipples. Your health care provider

Figure 23
Put a small amount of colostrum or
breastmilk on the nipple and areola after
each breastfeeding to ease soreness.

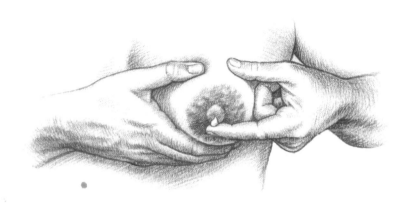

may suggest that you put a small amount of modified lanolin, a
glycerin gel pad, or a hydrogel dressing on the damaged area after
each breastfeeding to ease soreness and aid healing.

- Modified lanolin, Lansinoh, is a purified form of lanolin. It contains
  less pesticide residue and free lanolin alcohol than other lanolin
  products.

- Glycerin gel pads, Soothies, contain glycerin and water. Glycerin
  gel pads stay moist but will fill with fluid. If a pad gets thick and
  spongy, replace it with a new pad. Remove the pad before each
  feeding and reapply after.

- Hydrogel dressings are 96 percent water and come in solid sheets
  that can be cut to fit the size of the affected area. Hydrogel dressings dry out over time so you will need to replace the dressing
  every 1–3 days or as needed. Remove the dressing before each feeding and reapply after.

- If pain, cracking, or bleeding occurs, you can continue to breastfeed. But if breastfeeding is too painful, you can stop breastfeeding for 24 hours and let the nipple(s) heal. During this time, you will need to hand express or pump to relieve fullness. If only one breast is painful, continue to breastfeed on the healthy breast. If both breasts are painful, feed your baby your expressed breastmilk.

- Thick, yellow material draining from the damaged area can be a sign of infection and may require an antibiotic. Call your health care provider for help.

- A breast infection (*mastitis*) can occur when bacteria enter the breast through a break in the skin. Signs of infection include weakness, headache, nausea, soreness, chills, and fever (greater than 101° F or 38.4° C). A prescription medicine (antibiotic) may be necessary. If signs of mastitis occur, call your doctor right away. See "Mastitis (Breast Infection)," p. 61.

- If necessary, take acetaminophen or ibuprofen for pain and swelling.

To Prevent Sore Nipples

- Position your baby correctly on the breast. If necessary, hand express or pump to soften the breasts and relieve fullness.

- Breastfeed as long as your baby wishes on the first breast before offering the second breast.

- Begin each feeding on the breast offered last.

- Breastfeed every 1–3 hours during the day and every 2–3 hours at night. If you delay or skip feedings, hand express or pump to relieve fullness.

- Use the breastfeeding positions that are most comfortable for you and your baby (Figure 14, p. 23).

- Break the suction before removing your baby from the breast (Figure 17, p. 27).

Blisters

Signs

A collection of clear or bloody fluid underneath the skin.

Cause

A blister can form on the nipple or areola of the breast. Blisters are caused by friction or pressure on the skin while your baby breastfeeds. Blisters are usually filled with clear fluid but can be filled with blood. While the fluid can affect the taste of the milk, it will not hurt your baby. Because the fluid protects the new skin underneath, blisters should not be opened or drained. Leave them alone, and they will heal.

Recommended Treatment

- To soften the blister and prevent cracking, put warm water on the blistered area before each breastfeeding, using a towel or washcloth.

- Position your baby correctly on the breast (Figure 6, p. 11).

- Avoid breastfeeding positions that put pressure on the blistered area.

- If necessary, begin each feeding on the breast without the blister. When a let-down reflex occurs and milk begins to drip, switch to the breast with the blister.

- If necessary, limit the feeding time on the breast with the blister and breastfeed more often, every 1–2 hours.

To Prevent Blisters

- Position your baby correctly on the breast (Figure 6, p. 11).

- Use two or three different breastfeeding positions each day (Figure 14, p. 23).

- Hold your baby close to prevent unnecessary pulling on the breast.

- Offer both breasts at every feeding. Do not be concerned if your baby seems satisfied with one breast. If necessary, hand express or pump to relieve fullness in the second breast.

- Begin each feeding on the breast offered last.

Plugged Duct

Signs

Signs of a plugged duct include a red, tender area or a small lump in the breast. The lump may or may not be painful.

Cause

Narrow tubes (ducts) carry milk from the alveoli to the nipple openings. When feedings are delayed or missed, or when your baby breastfeeds poorly, milk can collect in the ducts and form a thick plug or small lump (Figure 24).

Recommended Treatment

- Put warm water on the plugged area before each breastfeeding.

- Breastfeed more often during the day.

- Begin each feeding on the breast with the plug.

- Adjust the position of your baby's mouth on the breast so that your baby's nose is pointing toward the plug.

- Gently massage the plugged area while your baby is feeding (Figure 22, p. 54).

- Hand express or pump after each breastfeeding to help remove the plug and relieve fullness.

- Choose a breastfeeding position that will best relieve fullness in the affected area.

- If a breast lump does not resolve within 2–3 days, call your doctor.

To Prevent Plugged Ducts

- Position your baby correctly on the breast.

- Use two or three different breastfeeding positions each day.

- Do not delay or skip feedings.

- If necessary, pump or hand express to relieve fullness.

- Avoid bras that are too tight or that bind, making it difficult to relieve fullness in all parts of the breast.

Figure 24
When breastfeedings are delayed or missed, or when your baby breastfeeds poorly, milk can collect in the ducts and form a thick plug or small lump.

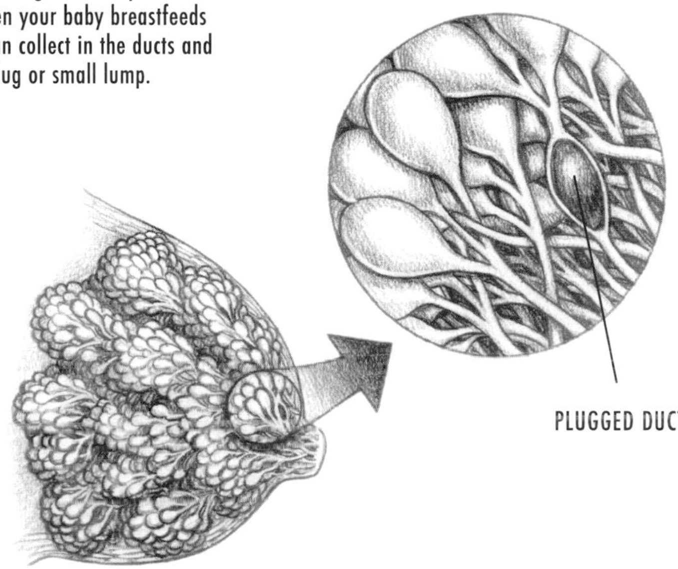

PLUGGED DUCT

Mastitis (Breast Infection)

Signs

There are two types of mastitis, infectious and noninfectious. Symptoms usually appear quickly and include weakness, headache, nausea, soreness, chills, and fever (greater than 101° F or 38.4° C). A portion of the breast may be red, hot, and painful.

Cause

A breast infection is usually caused by bacteria that enter the breast through an opening in the nipple or a break in the skin. Factors that increase the risk of a breast infection include cracked nipples, plugged ducts, infrequent or irregular breastfeedings or breast pumpings, tight-fitting bras, illness, fatigue, and stress.

Recommended Treatment

- Call your doctor. A prescription medicine (antibiotic) may be necessary. Although your symptoms may improve after 24–48 hours, take the medicine as directed until it is gone (usually 14 days).

- Put a warm pack on the infected area before each breastfeeding to aid let-down and relieve pain. Using a warm washcloth, taking a warm shower or tub bath, or soaking the breast in a pan of warm water works well.

- Continue to breastfeed frequently on both breasts. The infection will not harm your baby. Breastfeed every 1–3 hours during the day and every 2–3 hours at night.

- Start each feeding on the uninfected breast until a let-down reflex occurs, then switch to the infected breast. Breastfeed only until breast fullness is relieved and the breast softens. If necessary, hand express or pump to soften the breast and relieve fullness.

- You can apply cold packs after each breastfeeding to relieve pain and reduce swelling. Bags of frozen peas wrapped in a cold washcloth work well.

- Drink enough fluid to satisfy your thirst. Water and unsweetened fruit juices are best.

- Take acetaminophen or ibuprofen for pain and swelling.

- Get plenty of rest. Save time and energy by keeping your baby nearby.

To Prevent Mastitis

- Position your baby correctly on the breast (Figure 6, p. 11).

- If you delay or miss a feeding or if your baby breastfeeds poorly, hand express or pump to soften the breast and relieve fullness.

- Use two or three different breastfeeding positions each day (Figure 14, p. 23). This will help to relieve fullness in all parts of the breasts.

- Do not delay or skip feedings.

- Avoid bras that are too tight or that bind, making it difficult to relieve fullness in all parts of the breast.

- Wean gradually. Pump or hand express to relieve fullness and soften the breasts.

Fungal Infection (Candida Infection, Thrush)

Signs

Baby: Your baby can become infected during vaginal birth or while breastfeeding. Signs of infection often appear 2–4 weeks after birth and include small, white patches in the mouth (thrush) and/or a bright, red rash in the diaper area.

Mother: The mother can become infected while breastfeeding. Signs of infection include red or purple nipples, shiny areolas, and sharp, burning pain in the breast. Frequently the breasts look normal and severe pain is the only symptom. Some women also have a thick, white, vaginal discharge with redness, itching, and burning in the birth canal (*vagina*).

Father or sexual partner: Candida can spread easily from one family member to another through close contact. Your partner can become infected during sex. Signs of infection include a red rash on or around the penis and small white patches in the mouth.

Cause

Candida is a yeast-like fungus that grows in dark, damp places. It can be found in the birth canal and on the nipples and breasts of the mother as well as in the mouth and diaper area of the baby. Candida does not cause symptoms unless there is an overgrowth (too much). Because candida is found in the birth canal of most women, babies can become infected with candida during vaginal birth While the infection is seldom serious, it can be very painful. Sometimes an infected baby will refuse to breastfeed.

Recommended Treatment

- Both you and your baby need to be treated, even if only one of you has symptoms. This will prevent reinfection. You may need to call your doctor as well as your baby's doctor. In addition, treat your sexual partner or any other family member (e.g., your baby's siblings) who has signs of infection.

  Mother: Rinse your breasts with clear water after each breastfeeding. Your doctor can recommend an antifungal ointment such as Nystatin (mycostatin), Monistat (miconazole), Lotrimin (clotrimazole), or Bactroban (mupirocin). Put the ointment on the nipple and areola of both breasts after each breastfeeding for 14 days. If the pain is severe, your doctor can recommend a steroid ointment in addition to the anti-fungal ointment. Put a small amount of the steroid ointment on the nipples and areolas after each breastfeeding for 1–3 days; rub in well. It is not necessary to remove the ointment(s) before the next feeding.

Baby: Your baby's doctor can prescribe medication in liquid form for your baby's mouth and in ointment form for your baby's bottom. Paint the liquid on the inside of your baby's mouth (cheeks, gums, tongue, and roof) after each breastfeeding, using a clean cotton swab for each part of the mouth (Figure 25). If you put a used cotton swab back into the medicine bottle, you can transfer the fungus from your baby's mouth to the bottle. If your baby's symptoms include a red rash in the diaper area, apply an antifungal ointment during each diaper change.

- Change breast pads and diapers frequently. Do not use pads with plastic liners.

- Boil all nipples and pacifiers daily for 20 minutes. Replace with new ones after the first and second weeks of treatment.

- Wash bras in hot, soapy water each day and rinse well. Boil all pump parts for 20 minutes each day.

- Wash your hands carefully before each breastfeeding and after each diaper change.

- Use condoms during sex. Do not let your partner's mouth come into contact with your breasts.

- If signs of infection remain after 5–7 days of treatment, you may need to use a different medicine. Your doctor can suggest another ointment or he can recommend a 1 percent aqueous (water-based) solution of Gentian Violet. Apply the solution to the nipple and areola of both breasts and to the inside of your baby's mouth (cheeks, gums, tongue, and roof) using clean cotton swabs. Use sparingly—a little bit goes a long way. The purple solution will stain the skin and clothing so you might want to wear an old bra and T-shirt that can be thrown away. Apply the solution only once a day and for no more than 3 days. Gentian Violet can irritate your baby's mouth, so check with your baby's doctor before using Gentian Violet and discontinue its use right away if redness or sores appear.

- Resistant infections that do not respond to ointments or liquids can be treated with pills or tablets taken by mouth. Fluconazole (Diflucan) is approved by the Food and Drug Administration (FDA) for use in adults and infants. However, Diflucan should be used only if topical treatments (ointments and solutions) are ineffective. Discuss treatment options fully with your doctor and your baby's doctor. In addition, you may want to avoid foods that support the growth of fungus, such as alcohol, sugar, dairy products, wheat, nuts, peanut butter, dried fruits, and fruit juices.

To Prevent Fungal Infections

- Wash your hands carefully before each breastfeeding and after each diaper change. Remove artificial nails where fungus can grow.

- Change breast pads and diapers frequently. Do not use pads with plastic liners.

- Avoid the daily use of creams and lotions. They keep the skin moist but may encourage the growth of yeast-like fungus or bacteria.

- Keep your nipples uncovered as much as possible. You can open the flaps on your nursing bra or remove your bra for periods of time each day and at night.

Figure 25
Use a clean cotton swab for each part of your baby's mouth (roof, cheeks, tongue, gums) when treating for thrush.

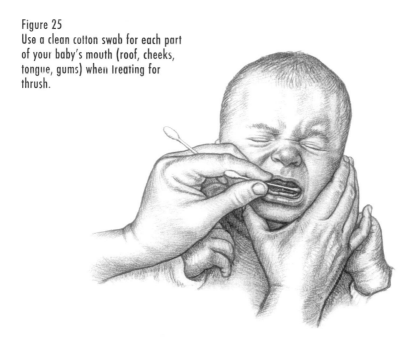

Leaking

Signs

You may feel a tingling sensation just before your milk starts to drip or spray. Or you may simply notice a wet spot on your clothing.

Cause

Leaking is caused by the let-down reflex. When your baby breastfeeds, milk often drips or sprays from the other breast. Leaking can also occur between feedings. Although leaking is common, it does not occur in all mothers. Leaking occurs more often during the early weeks when your baby's breastfeeding schedule is constantly changing. Once your baby has a set feeding schedule (at about 6–12 weeks of age), your milk supply will vary less from day to day and you will have less leaking. Leaking can also occur when you think about your baby, when you hear your baby or another baby cry, when you delay or skip a feeding and your breasts overfill, or when you are making love and have an orgasm (sexual climax). Even a warm shower can cause a let-down reflex to occur and milk to leak.

Recommended Treatment

- Use breast pads to provide short-term protection for your clothing. Breast pads come in all shapes and sizes. They can be disposable or reusable. You can even make your own pads using cloth diapers, cotton fabric, or men's handkerchiefs. Change pads frequently. Do not use pads with waterproof liners.

- Choose clothing with light colors and small prints that will cover up a multitude of mishaps.

- Place a bath towel on top of the bed sheet. This will protect the mattress and keep the bed linens dry.

- Keep an extra nightgown handy just in case.

- Breastfeed your baby before making love or going to bed. This will limit the amount of milk in the breasts and allow time for sex or sleep, whichever comes first!

- Press firmly against the nipple of each breast with the palm of your hand or your wrist, or fold your arms tightly across your chest, in order to slow the leaking. It is best to limit this practice in the early weeks as it can interfere with the let-down reflex and may decrease your milk supply.

To Prevent Leaking

Leaking lets you know that you are making milk. Leaking also helps to increase your confidence in your ability to breastfeed. If you try to prevent leaking, you may find that your milk supply stays low. So keep breast pads handy and allow your breasts to drip, drip, drip!

9 Breastfeeding After a Cesarean Birth

Cesarean birth, often called a "C-section," is the surgical removal of the baby through an incision or opening made in the mother's abdomen. About 20–30 percent of all births are cesarean births. Cesarean births are seldom planned; as a result, parents may experience many feelings including anger, relief, frustration, joy, and sadness. Discuss your feelings openly with your doctor, family, or friends. It may help to talk with other parents who have had an unplanned cesarean birth. While a cesarean birth will not affect your ability to produce milk, pain and weakness may make it necessary for you to depend on others for help. If you or your baby needs special care, the start of breastfeeding may be delayed.

In the Hospital

- Breastfeed as soon as possible after birth.

- If the start of breastfeeding is delayed for more than 24–48 hours, begin expressing your milk. The goal of early, frequent milk expression is to let your body know that a lot of milk will be needed in a few days. See Chapter 19, "Expression and Collection of Human Milk," for information on expressing milk. A fully automatic electric pump with a double collection kit that lets you pump both breasts at the same time works best (Figure 26)

- Choose a comfortable position for breastfeeding (Figure 14, p. 23). Use extra pillows to protect the incision and provide support.

- Position your baby correctly on the breast (see Figure 6, p. 11). You may need help with positioning, turning, and burping (babies born by cesarean birth often have more mucus).

- Breastfeed whenever your baby seems fussy or hungry (about 8–12 times in each 24 hours). Expect to breastfeed every 1–3 hours during the day and every 2–3 hours at night. Breastfeed as long as your baby wishes on the first breast before offering the second breast.

- Increase the amount of protein (meat, fish, milk, eggs, tofu) and fiber (whole grains, raw vegetables) in your diet.

- Drink to satisfy your thirst. Warm liquids will get your bladder and bowel working again.

- Take short, frequent walks. Mild exercise increases bowel activity and helps you regain your strength.

- Get plenty of rest. If necessary, limit phone calls and visitors.

- Pain medicine may be necessary for several days. Your doctor will prescribe medicine that is safe for you and your baby.

Figure 26
A fully automatic electric pump with a double collection kit lets you pump both breasts at the same time. (Examples shown are Lactina by Medela and Elite by Ameda/Hollister.)

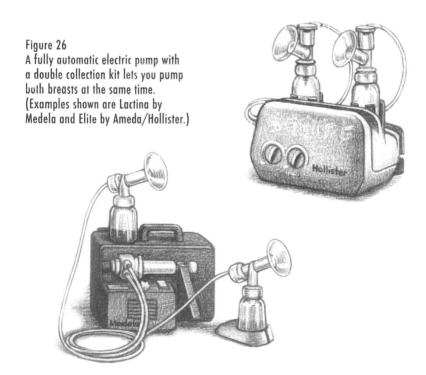

At Home

- Breastfeed whenever your baby seems fussy or hungry (about 8–12 times in each 24 hours). Expect to breastfeed every 1–3 hours during the day and every 2–3 hours at night. Some babies will not ask to eat often enough. During the first 2–4 weeks, if your baby does not wake frequently to breastfeed, you may need to watch for early signs of hunger or light sleep. Signs of hunger can include sucking sounds, sucking movements, squirming, coughing, and yawning. Offer the breast when you see these signs.

- Keep your baby in the room with you to save time and energy.

- Get plenty of rest. Nap when your baby naps.

- Limit your activity. Avoid heavy lifting, household chores, and brisk exercise for 4–6 weeks.

- To promote healing and speed recovery, continue to:

  - eat a high-protein, high-fiber diet

  - drink enough liquids to satisfy your thirst

  - get mild to moderate exercise

The birth of a tiny baby born weeks or months premature can be scary.

"Why did this happen?"

"Was it something I did?"

"Was it something I didn't do?"

"Will he live?"

"Will he be normal?"

"How long will he be in the hospital?"

"Can I hold him?"

"How will he eat if he is too little to suck?"

"Can I breastfeed?"

Premature babies can be breastfed even if they need special care. Breastfeeding gives parents a chance to share in the care of their baby, to do something that no one else can do, to parent in a very special way. If your baby is too small or too sick to breastfeed in the beginning, he can still be fed your breastmilk.

Even when you give birth prematurely, your milk contains just the right amount of nutrients to meet your baby's needs. In addition, human milk contains special cells that protect babies against infections, which are common in premature babies. Breastmilk is easy to digest, which is important for premature babies with immature digestive systems. Also, research shows that premature babies who are fed human milk for at least the first month of life have a higher intelligence quotient (IQ) at ages 7–8 years than babies fed infant formula.

Let your baby's doctor and nurses know as soon as possible that you plan to breastfeed. The hospital staff can give you information on milk production as well as the expression, collection, and storage of breastmilk. In addition, they can put you in touch with other parents who have breastfed premature babies. These parents, along with the medical team, can help you develop realistic goals and provide you with much-needed encouragement and support. As your baby's condition improves and your confidence in your ability to care for your baby grows, you will be glad you chose to breastfeed.

Breastfeeding even a healthy, full-term infant can be a challenge, and breastfeeding a premature baby can be overwhelming at times. If you get discouraged, you may find it helpful to know that premature babies benefit even more from human milk than full-term babies do.

Early Feedings

Your baby may be too small or too sick to breastfeed in the beginning and will need to be fed a special liquid through a small tube or needle that is placed in one of his veins (*intravenous* feeding). As his condition improves, he will be fed your breastmilk through a small tube that is passed through his nose and into his stomach (*gavage* feeding).

Milk Expression

- If your baby is unable to breastfeed, you should begin pumping as soon as possible after birth. Unless you are very sick, it is important to start pumping within 24–48 hours. The goal of early, frequent milk expression is to let your body know that a lot of milk will be needed soon.

- Ask your nurse for a fully automatic electric pump to use while you are in the hospital (Figure 27). Even if your baby is able to breastfeed, you may want to use a semi-automatic, battery-operated, or hand pump to increase your milk supply.

- Your expressed colostrum or breastmilk can be collected and fed to your baby or frozen and used later. If your baby needs to stay in the

Figure 27
If your baby is too small or too sick to breastfeed, you can use a fully automatic electric pump while you are in the hospital. (Examples shown are Lact-e by Ameda/Hollister and Symphony by Medela.)

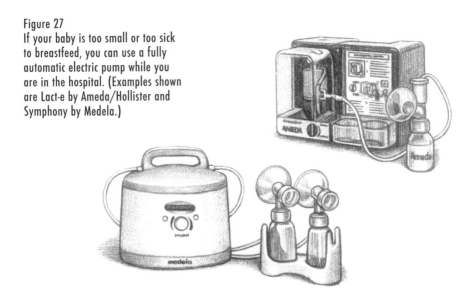

hospital for many days or weeks, you can rent or purchase a fully automatic electric pump to use when you go home.

- Each time you pump and before you handle the pump parts, wash your hands with soap and water and rinse well.

- Follow the directions for expressing with a breast pump in Chapter 19, p. 143.

- Pump *at least* eight times in each 24 hours for about 20–30 minutes each time. You will need to pump every 2–4 hours during the day and every 4–6 hours at night when awake. Many mothers pump every 3 hours during the day and sleep for 6 hours at night. Since pumps never get tired, hungry, or full, think of pumping as a special time to relax, think about your baby, and "feed" him. If you pump just before you go to bed, you will be able to sleep comfortably for a longer period of time.

- Many mothers get more milk with the first pumping session than with the next three or four, and then the amount slowly increases over the next several days. By the end of the first week, you should be getting at least 1 ounce from each breast during each pumping session. If necessary, talk with the lactation consultant or your doctor about ways to increase your milk supply.

■ During the first week, as your breasts change from making colostrum to making mature milk, they may feel very full. You will need to pump more to relieve the fullness and stay comfortable. This will help you build a good milk supply that can adjust to your baby's needs later as he grows. Though you may be making more milk than your baby needs, if you do not relieve the fullness and soften your breasts, you may never have the full supply of milk that your baby will need later. When the breasts stay full, your body will respond by making less milk.

■ Plan to do some relaxation exercises at least once a day even if you cannot do them just before pumping.

■ If you are able to pump in the hospital, sit next to your baby's crib, cot, or isolette; hold his hand if possible. If you are at home, make a phone call to the nursery to check on your baby's condition.

Milk Storage

Because freezing affects the anti-infective properties of breastmilk, it is best to provide fresh, unfrozen breastmilk each day if possible. Store your expressed milk in clean containers provided by the nursery. Glass or hard plastic containers with solid lids are recommended. Label each container with your baby's name, your name, the date, and the time the milk was collected. If you are taking any medicine, write the name of the medicine on the label.

Ask your baby's nurse how much he is being fed each 24 hours and store your milk in 24-hour portions or single servings to prevent waste. If your baby is very small or not gaining weight, and you are pumping more than twice what he is being fed, pump the foremilk and freeze it for later use. Then pump the hindmilk to take to the nursery.

The composition of stored human milk is affected by time and temperature. Recommended storage times are based on current research; however, research results vary. So, in the interest of safety, human milk intended for sick or premature babies should be refrigerated right away if possible.

When refrigeration is not readily available, human milk can be stored at room temperature (25°C or 77°F) for up to 5 hours. It can be stored in a refrigerator (4°C or 39°F) for up to 5 days, in the freezer section of a refrigerator/freezer (-5°C or 23°F) for up to 5 months, or in an upright or chest freezer (-20°C or -4°F) for up to 12 months (Figure 28).

Place all containers in the middle of the refrigerator or freezer section to prevent warming when the door is opened and closed. Storage has little effect on the protein and carbohydrate in human milk, but changes in the fat can give the milk a soapy taste, so always use the oldest milk first.

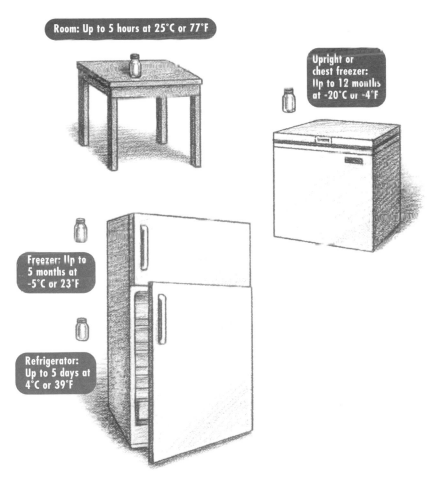

Figure 28
Breastmilk storage guidelines for premature babies.

Table 4. Human Milk Storage Recommendations for Premature Babies*

HUMAN MILK	ROOM TEMPERATURE (25°C OR 77°F)	REFRIGERATOR (4°C OR 39°F)	FREEZER SECTION (-5°C OR 23°F)	UPRIGHT OR CHEST FREEZER (-20°C OR -4°F)
Fresh	Use within 5 hours	Use within 5 days	Use within 5 months	Use within 12 months
Previously frozen, then thawed in refrigerator	Use within 4 hours	Use within 24 hours	Do not refreeze	Do not refreeze
Previously frozen, then thawed in warm water	Use right away	Use within 4 hours	Do not refreeze	Do not refreeze

* Fresh breastmilk is best for your baby.

Getting to Know Your Baby as His Condition Improves

As soon as your baby is stable and can be held for a period of time each day, ask his nurse if you can place him underneath your clothing and cuddle him skin-to-skin against your chest (kangaroo care). This early contact gives mothers and fathers a chance to care for their baby and to gain confidence in their ability to parent (Figure 29). Safe and secure against your chest, your baby receives all the warmth he needs as he gets to know you. Plan to hold him like this for about an hour at a time. The most stressful time for your baby is when he is being taken out of or put in the isolette, not the time he spends sleeping on your chest.

Both mothers and fathers can provide kangaroo care. Babies who are held skin-to-skin gain weight faster, move into an open crib sooner, and go home earlier. Also, mothers who provide kangaroo care often breastfeed for longer periods of time. You may notice that your breasts leak while you are holding your baby skin to skin, and that you are able to pump more milk after providing kangaroo care.

Beginning to Breastfeed a Premature Baby

Talk with the medical staff about your baby's readiness to breastfeed. Recent studies suggest that a baby's ability to suck, swallow, and breathe in an organized manner is the best indication of readiness to breastfeed and may appear as soon as 32 weeks' gestation. Many babies can breastfeed, without showing signs of stress, days or weeks before they can bottle-feed.

Once your baby is ready to breastfeed, ask for (or bring from home) a pillow to support him at your breast. The football hold or cross-cradle hold usually works best in the beginning (Figure 14, p. 23). Loosen your baby's blanket so his arms can hug your breast. Support his back, shoulders, and head in the palm of your hand. His ear, shoulder, and hip should be in a straight line so his jaw can relax to open. Express a few drops of breastmilk onto your nipple and areola.

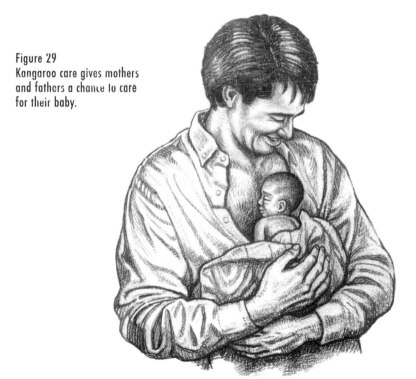

Figure 29
Kangaroo care gives mothers and fathers a chance to care for their baby.

Support your breast with your other hand and shape the areola and nipple into a wedge. Gently touch your baby's nose with your nipple. As he opens his mouth, continue holding your breast as you hug him to the breast. Resist the urge to press on his head, because that will make it difficult for him to swallow and breathe. "Dancer hand" support is helpful for tiny babies with weak muscles (Figure 30). Using your thumb and first finger to form a U shape, support your baby's chin on the breast with your hand.

If your milk is flowing freely, your baby may just lick and swallow. If your milk flows more slowly, he will start to suckle and swallow. He should suckle in bursts of at least six suckle/swallows (some babies do many more) and then will pause before he suckles again. As he slows down, you can massage or compress the breast to move more hindmilk into his mouth (Figure 22, p. 54). Remember that he has never had to *eat* before—the milk was just dripped into his stomach—so he may not be really eager right away.

Figure 30
"Dancer hand" support can
be helpful for tiny babies
with weak muscles.

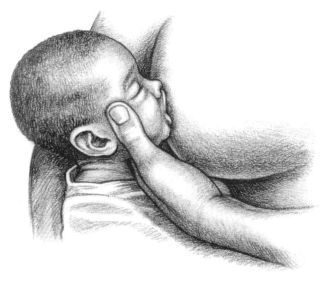

These first breastfeedings are a learning experience for both you and your baby, so relax and enjoy each moment. If you do not hear your baby swallow and your breast does not soften, his nurse can give him your breastmilk through a feeding tube (gavage feeding).

Often a mother is making more milk than her baby can take at first. If you are pumping 2–3 ounces per pumping session and your baby is being fed only 1 ounce per feeding, expect that he will soften only one breast. You will need to pump when you finish holding him. You may find that after your baby has breastfed you can pump more milk than usual for that time of day. Until your baby is fully breastfeeding, continue to pump after each feeding to soften your breasts.

If you are pumping more than twice what your baby is taking per feeding, pump one breast partially and then breastfeed on that breast. This will ensure that your baby is getting the higher-calorie hindmilk, which will help him grow faster.

At first your baby may be able to breastfeed only once every 24 hours. The rest of his feedings will still be through a tube while he sleeps. Soon he will be ready for two breastfeedings a day, usually separated by at least one or two tube feedings.

When your baby is ready for a third breastfeeding each day, you will want to talk to the medical staff about doing two breastfeedings in a row to save you time and to see if your baby has the energy to feed at the breast twice in a row. As he gets closer to coming home, he may start to gag on the feeding tube, which is a sign that he is maturing. A feeding tube can be put through his nose and left there between feedings, or he can be fed with a cup or bottle.

Timing of Feedings

Premature babies go through several feeding patterns as they approach full term. If your baby is very small, he may start out with a continuous drip of milk into his stomach. Gradually a larger amount of milk is given every 3 hours—the same pattern as for a breastfeeding baby.

Then, often at about 34–35 weeks' gestation, babies seem to be able to eat more at one time, but they awaken less frequently. If it is very difficult to wake your baby for feedings every 3 hours, talk with his doctor or nurse about moving him to a 4-hour schedule for a while. Expect that when he comes home he will change back to a 3-hour schedule as he gets closer to his due date. That is another sign that he is maturing. Since he is staying awake longer and getting more active, he needs to eat more often.

Providing a Supplement/Substitute

Your milk supply may be low despite regular pumping, and breastmilk (your frozen milk or banked donor milk) or formula supplements may be necessary. If you follow each breastfeeding with a bottle-feeding, some babies can become confused. Milk flows faster from a bottle than from a breast, and bottle-feeding takes less effort than breastfeeding. So your baby may learn to like bottle-feeding more than breastfeeding.

If you need to give your baby a supplement, you can use a supplemental feeding device while you are breastfeeding (Figure 31). A supplemental feeding device is a plastic container, filled with human milk or formula, which hangs on a cord around the mother's neck. A thin piece of plastic tubing stretches from the top of the container to the nipple of each breast, where the tubing is taped into place. When your baby breastfeeds, he receives milk from the breast and supplement from the container.

Once your baby is breastfeeding well and a good milk supply is established, the supplement can be discontinued. To ease your mind, you can weigh your baby before and after feedings using a special scale. If breastmilk production remains low, talk with a lactation consultant, doctor, or nurse about ways to increase your milk supply.

Figure 31
You can supplement your baby at the
breast using a supplemental feeding device.
(Example shown is a Supplemental Nursing
System by Medela.)

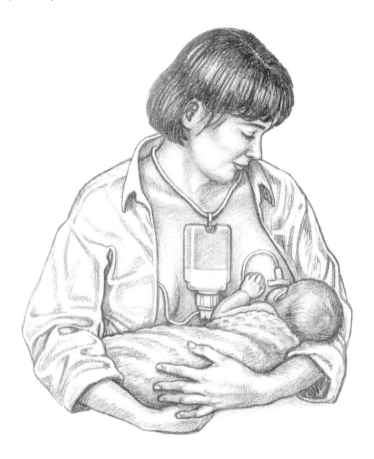

11 Breastfeeding More Than One Baby

You can produce enough milk to totally meet the nutritional needs of two (or more) babies. The amount of milk you make depends on the amount removed from your breasts during breastfeedings or through milk expression. Early, frequent breastfeedings—or milk expression, if one or more babies need special care—will help you get off to the best possible start.

All the advantages of breastfeeding for mother and babies are multiplied when you give birth to two or more babies. Your babies benefit from the perfect blend of nutrients and anti-infective properties that breastmilk provides. You benefit from the release of oxytocin that limits uterine bleeding, which can be greater after a multiple birth. You and your partner will appreciate the fact that breastfeeding requires little or no preparation and also offers cost savings. All will benefit from the enforced skin-to-skin contact that can help you get to know each baby as an individual.

Planning Ahead

Be prepared to begin breastfeeding under many different circumstances. Surgical (cesarean) birth, preterm delivery, and other conditions resulting in a need for special care for one or more babies are more common with multiple births.

- Attend childbirth preparation and surgical birth classes early in pregnancy, beginning in your fourth or fifth month.

- Share and discuss information about breastfeeding multiples with your partner, family, and friends.

- Locate resources for buying or renting a breast pump should milk expression be necessary. Pumps can be rented or purchased from hospitals, pump rental stations, and medical supply companies.

- Contact a breastfeeding support group such as La Leche League or a support group for parents of multiples such as a Mothers of Twins club. Ask if someone can put you in touch with another mother who has successfully breastfed the same number of multiples as you will be having.

- Choose a pediatrician, family practice physician, or pediatric nurse practitioner who is knowledgeable about breastfeeding and who has cared for successfully breastfed multiples.

- Ask your partner, a family member, or a friend to stay with you at night while you are in the hospital, so that you will have extra help when you begin to breastfeed your babies.

- Arrange for daily or round-the-clock household help for several weeks after your babies come home from the hospital.

- Set a goal to continue breastfeeding for at least 6–8 weeks after birth, no matter how difficult it may seem at times.

The encouragement and support of those close to you, another breastfeeding mother of multiples, and your babies' health care provider will give you confidence in your ability to produce all that your babies need.

Beginning to Breastfeed

Healthy, full-term multiples. Ideally, your babies' first breastfeeding will occur soon after birth. Healthy infants born at, or close to, full term usually search for and crawl to their mother's breast within an hour of birth. Although rooming-in, or a modified version of it, is possible with twins, you may need the help of a family member or friend if you have a surgical delivery or triplets. It is easier to breastfeed frequently when babies are accessible, and your confidence in handling them can grow when a nurse or a lactation consultant is available.

When rooming-in is not possible, ask that all babies be brought to you for all feedings. Each multiple is a single baby needing 8–12 breastfeedings in a 24-hour period. In the beginning, it may seem confusing if each baby has a somewhat different, although normal, breastfeeding pattern. Until you have a better sense of each baby's breastfeeding style, it may help to write down feedings and wet and dirty diapers on a checklist that is color-coded for each multiple.

Preterm or sick multiples. When preterm or sick multiples need to stay in a neonatal intensive care unit (NICU), you will want to begin expressing your milk within 24–48 hours of giving birth, if your condition permits. See Chapter 19, "Expression and Collection of Human Milk," for detailed information on expressing milk.

If you are sick and unable to express milk on your own, a nurse, lactation consultant, family member, or friend can help you use a breast pump. Do not worry about the quantity of milk you express. The goal of early, frequent milk expression is to let your body know that a lot of milk will be needed in a short time. The sooner and more often you express your breastmilk, the sooner you will produce greater amounts of milk.

Most mothers find it easier to manage frequent milk expression if they use a fully automatic electric pump. When a double collection kit is used, it is possible to save time by pumping both breasts at once (Figure 26, p. 69). Double-pumping also increases prolactin levels, which increases milk production.

Begin by pumping at least eight times a day. Pump *at least* eight times in each 24 hours for about 20–30 minutes each time. You will need to pump every 2–4 hours during the day and every 4–6 hours at night when awake. Many mothers pump every 3 hours during the day and sleep for 6 hours at night. To increase milk production for multiples, increase the number of pumping sessions as your babies' condition improves or any time you notice a decline in breastmilk volume. Many mothers find that their milk production varies with the condition of their babies. By the time your babies begin to breastfeed, you will want to be pumping 8–12 times in each 24 hours.

Sometimes one (or more) of your babies is able to room in with you. Or one is discharged earlier, while the other(s) must remain in the NICU. In this situation, breastfeed each baby who is with you 8–12 times in 24 hours. You can pump for any multiple(s) in the NICU. To save time, pump one breast while one baby breastfeeds on the other breast. If you don't think you are ready to coordinate pumping with breastfeeding, pump both breasts immediately after a breastfeeding, or pump between breastfeedings.

Multiples with feeding difficulties. Multiples, including those born at or close to full term, are more likely to experience pregnancy, labor, and birth situations that can influence their initial ability to latch on and breastfeed correctly. One multiple may be affected more than the other(s). In addition, some preterm or sick multiples have difficulty making the transition to the breast because of exposure to other feeding methods that interfere with oral behaviors needed for effective breastfeeding. For example, the use of a bottle and an artificial nipple may interfere with the tongue placement and movement needed for breastfeeding.

These types of feeding difficulties may last from several hours to several weeks, but they tend to be short-lived. Most can be resolved with patience and persistence. However, "short-lived" may seem like forever when you are sleep-deprived and juggling breastfeedings, supplemental feedings, and breast pumping sessions. Contact a breastfeeding mothers' support group and/or an International Board Certified Lactation Consultant (IBCLC) to help you. A support group or IBCLC can offer practical problem-solving strategies and provide moral support.

Developing a Feeding Routine

Almost any method of coordinating breastfeedings will work as long as each baby breastfeeds 8–12 times in 24 hours. Some mothers breastfeed each baby on both breasts at every feeding. However, many mothers find it less confusing to feed one baby on only one breast at each feeding. This also makes it possible to breastfeed two babies at the same time. If you let each baby breastfeed as long as desired, so that your babies, not you, choose when to end a feeding, your milk supply will quickly increase to meet your babies' needs.

To stimulate milk production equally in both breasts, it is a good idea to alternate babies and breasts. You may alternate babies and breasts for each feeding, but many mothers find it is easier to alternate babies and breasts on a daily basis. For example, today Baby A (and Baby C) feeds on the right breast and Baby B (and Baby D) on the left. Then tomorrow Baby A (and Baby C) feeds on the left breast and Baby B (and Baby D) on the right.

Mothers of odd-numbered multiples may have to alternate babies and breasts more often than every 24 hours. If you feed the baby who wakes first, you probably will find that the one(s) feeding second on a breast, and last, will be the one(s) ready to eat first at the next feeding.

Some mothers assign babies a specific breast. Milk production in each breast then adapts to that individual baby's needs. However, you may find yourself with breasts of very different sizes! Also, you may find another multiple unwilling to breastfeed on the unfamiliar side if a situation arises in which one baby cannot breastfeed for a period of time, such as during a nursing strike (see "What are nursing strikes?" on p. 168), which is more common with multiples than with single-birth infants. If you choose to have each baby always feed at a specific breast, vary feeding positions from feeding to feeding.

Breastfeeding simultaneously (two babies at once) can save a lot of time. Some mothers always breastfeed two; others never breastfeed simultaneously. Most mothers do both. They simultaneously feed two for some feedings and feed the babies separately for others. It usually depends on the babies' and mother's needs during any given feeding.

Don't begin simultaneous feedings until you feel comfortable positioning and helping a single baby latch on to the breast. At least one baby should be able to latch on and breastfeed without difficulty before you attempt to feed two at once. If both infants demonstrate any incorrect breastfeeding behaviors, simultaneous feedings may reinforce those behaviors.

Even if you or the babies find simultaneous feeding difficult to master in the early weeks, keep trying. It usually becomes much easier after several weeks or a few months when babies have become skilled at latching on to the breast. Use pillows to hold babies in position so that your hands are free to help with latch-on. Many mothers prefer the support of a firm breastfeeding pillow. You may want to work with pillows already available in your home before purchasing a special pillow, since some mothers find that pillows with a little "give" are more useful for positioning babies.

The following positions are the ones used most often for simultaneous breastfeedings (Figure 32).

Double-football/double-clutch hold. In this position, a baby's body is tucked under each of your arms (or is supported on a pillow at your side) while a baby's head is supported in each of your hands (or on a pillow). A mother's hands are free to help babies latch on when pillows are used to hold babies in place, so many mothers learn this position first. This position also limits pressure on the incision area after a surgical birth. However, it can be the least "hands-on" position, which is a disadvantage because it limits your ability to touch your baby.

Criss-cross/double-cradle hold. With a baby's head cradled in the bend of each arm and the babies' chests rolled to face your chest, criss-cross the babies' bodies in front of your abdomen. A pillow on your lap and under each elbow often adds comfort and support. You may be more comfortable if you place your feet on a stool, sit in a recliner, or tailor-sit (cross-legged) on the floor. This position increases skin-to-skin contact between mothers and babies and enhances baby-to-baby contact.

Some mothers adjust this position with older babies by cradling each baby's head and supporting a baby's body parallel to each of the mother's legs. To breastfeed in bed, a mother can lie on her back, and, with a baby's head cradled in each arm, lay a baby's body along each arm, parallel to each side of her abdomen. The babies' heads and bodies are rolled toward and face each breast.

Combination cradle-football/layered/parallel hold(s). With Baby A held in the traditional cradle hold, Baby B's head is supported in your hand or on a pillow or "layered" gently on Baby A's abdomen. Tuck Baby B's body under your arm or lay his body on a pillow out to the side at a right angle from your body. This position lends itself better to discreet breastfeeding. It is a "hands-on" position, yet one or both hands can be free to help assist with latch-on.

Figure 32
Breastfeeding multiples simultaneously
saves time and energy.

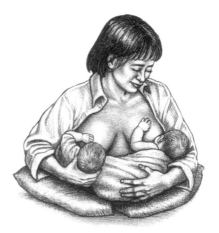

**COMBINATION CRADLE-FOOTBALL/
LAYERED/PARALLEL HOLDS**

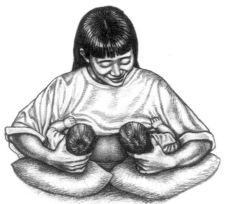

DOUBLE-FOOTBALL/DOUBLE-CLUTCH HOLD

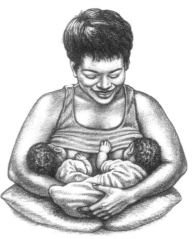

CRISS-CROSS/DOUBLE-CRADLE HOLD

Partially Breastfeeding

Full or nearly full breastfeeding is ideal for babies, but it may not always be possible with multiples. Partial breastfeeding provides babies with varying degrees of nutritional and anti-infective benefits. The benefits depend on the number of breastfeedings (or amount of breast-milk) each receives. Regardless of the amount of breastmilk provided, research indicates that any amount of breastfeeding, or breastmilk, is much better than none.

Mothers choose partial breastfeeding for a variety of reasons. Sometimes they want some relief with feedings. Often partial breast-feeding is chosen because of ongoing feeding difficulties. Others choose partial breastfeeding when they return to work outside the home. Some mothers partially breastfeed, but their babies still receive only breastmilk. These mothers pump their breasts once or twice a day, and their babies then receive the expressed milk from a bottle or cup.

Because breastfeeding means more than good nutrition to babies and mothers, fully breastfeeding one (or more) and fully bottle-feeding the other(s) should be avoided if at all possible. It may lead to long-lasting differences in a mother's feelings for her babies. In the rare instances when it is necessary, mothers should be aware of this concern and increase skin-to-skin contact with any bottle-fed baby.

Combining Breastfeeding and Bottle-Feeding

Partial breastfeeding is more successful when bottles are offered on a limited basis. To maintain adequate milk production and avoid unantici-pated weaning, breastfeed at least 8–12 times each day. For example, breastfeed each twin at least four to six times in each 24 hours, each triplet at least three or four times, and each quadruplet at least two or three times. Remaining feedings can be expressed breastmilk or infant formula if breastmilk is not available.

Most mothers choose to offer a bottle during the night or in the evening when babies tend to cluster-feed. You can breastfeed first, then ask your partner to offer each baby a bottle to complement, or "top off," an evening feeding. Other options include your partner bottle-feeding one (or more) while you breastfeed the other(s), or your part-ner bottle-feeding all babies during one nighttime feeding while you breastfeed all during the next feeding.

Breastmilk-Feeding

Mothers sometimes choose to exclusively bottle-feed expressed breast-milk (*breastmilk-feed*) when one or more babies experience an ongoing difficulty at the breast. Short-term breastmilk feeding can give a mother a chance to focus on increasing or maintaining milk production when breast pumping, breastfeedings, and supplemental feedings have become overwhelming. There are mothers who breastmilk-feed for longer periods. Some choose to continue pumping 8–12 times a day for many months and offer the expressed milk in a bottle or cup.

Returning to Work

Employed mothers of multiples usually find it easier to continue breast-feeding when they rent or purchase a fully automatic electric pump with a double collection kit. Try to pump every 2–3 hours while away from your babies. If you want your babies to receive only your breast-milk for their first 6 months, you may have to schedule one or two additional 10- to 15-minute pumping sessions each day to maintain adequate milk production.

Maintaining Perspective

Each of your multiple babies has the same needs as any single-birth infant, so multiples require more time and effort no matter how they are fed. Remembering this may help on those days when you feel as if you have competed in a breastfeeding marathon and have just "hit the wall." When you wonder if you will ever experience the "joys" of breastfeeding, it can help to recall that your babies have been enjoying the benefits of breastfeeding and breastmilk from day one.

Your multiples will be breastfeeding babies for only a brief period of time. Maintain perspective by accepting all offers of help, surrounding yourself with a supportive network of family and friends, and finding the humor amid the chaos! Confidence in your body's ability to make enough milk, and in your babies' ability to get all they need through breastfeeding, will grow as your babies grow. Before you know it, you will be numbering yourself among the many mothers who have suc-cessfully breastfed multiples.

12

Breastfeeding an Adopted or Previously Weaned Baby

In a culture where many women have doubts about their ability to produce enough milk for their babies, it may seem impossible to consider:

- *relactation*—reestablishing a milk supply that has disappeared, or nearly so, or

- *induced lactation*—establishing a milk supply without a prior pregnancy.

Yet many women all over the world have been able to breastfeed their babies—both "homemade" and adopted— in these ways.

To understand how it is possible to relactate or induce lactation, you will want to refer back to pp. 6–14. To relactate or induce lactation, you need the same three ingredients you need in the more usual breastfeeding situation: a breast, a baby, and a brain.

A baby's sucking stimulates the pituitary gland to release both prolactin (the milk-producing hormone) and oxytocin (the hormone that releases milk).

If this stimulation is repeated often enough, the alveoli (the milk-producing cells in the breast) will begin to do what they are designed to do—make milk.

Continued stimulation will cause the muscles surrounding the alveoli to contract and move any milk there through the milk ducts to the nipple openings so that it can be transferred to the baby.

It is as simple as that—in theory. In practice it is a bit more complicated. Because breastfeeding is a partnership between a mother and her baby, both of them need to be actively involved in the process. If a mother has little or no milk, her baby may be unwilling to breastfeed. And if a baby is being fed artificially, especially with a bottle, his interest in breastfeeding may be very low. The mother attempting to relactate or induce lactation must find a way to do all of the following:

- Encourage her baby to latch on to the breast and suckle effectively.

- Ensure that her baby is being adequately nourished while she is building a milk supply.

- Maintain the special mother-child bond.

- Maintain her own interest and enthusiasm for breastfeeding.

Why Relactate (or Induce Lactation)?

The usual benefits for both mother and child—physical, emotional, social, and economic—outlined on pp. 1–5 apply when a mother relactates for her homemade baby. Many of the benefits also apply to adoptive breastfeeding, but because lactating in this situation takes special effort, it is helpful to review the benefits and ask which are especially important to you.

With both relactation and induced lactation, the long-term benefits are likely to outweigh the short-term benefits. In addition, the emotional benefits may be more apparent than the physical benefits—especially in the early days.

Some mothers need to wean sooner than they had planned. A mother and baby may be separated because of illness or other causes. Many mothers relactate because they want their babies to have the nutritional and immunological benefits of human milk. In some cases, mothers find after weaning that their babies can tolerate only their breastmilk, and reestablishing a milk supply is a high priority.

Mothers establishing a milk supply for an adopted baby often do so because they know that breastfeeding promotes the development of the special bond between a mother and her child—a bond that would, with a homemade baby, already have begun during pregnancy.

Nutritional and immunological benefits tend to be dose-related. While even a small amount of breastmilk is valuable, the baby who receives large amounts has more optimal nutrition and better long- and short-term protection against a variety of illnesses. Until a mother is producing significant quantities of milk, these benefits will probably not figure as prominently among her priorities.

Getting Started

Getting started may be as simple as just putting your baby to the breast and seeing what happens. Young babies—and especially those who have had some experience at the breast—are more likely to be the ones who figure out what to do right away and suck at the breast as though they have been breastfeeding all their young lives. Don't assume that your baby is going to have difficulty just because he is a little older. Many older babies also take to the breast surprisingly well—even without prior experience.

Some babies may need a little help to latch on correctly (see pp. 24–27); others may need encouragement to even try.

Helping Your Baby to Take the Breast

If your baby is having trouble latching on to the breast or seems reluctant to try, he will need a little extra encouragement. The following strategies have been helpful to other mothers.

- Keep your baby in close, skin-to-skin contact. Kangaroo care (see p. 76) will help your baby get acquainted with you through his senses –smell, touch, taste, hearing, and sight—and, in addition, stimulates your body to release prolactin.

- Give your baby a chance to repeat the experience he had—or might have had—right after birth. Place him skin-to-skin on your abdomen just below your breasts. Stroke him and talk to him gently and let him explore at his own pace. Encourage him to seek your breast. As long as his inborn reflex to do so is still intact, there is a good chance that he will slowly make his way to your breast and latch on.

- Try taking a bath with your baby. Many babies who have difficulty latching on to the breast do better in a warm water bath. After one or two in-water attachments, your baby can usually practice his new skill on "dry land."

■ Even during those times when your baby is not in skin-to-skin contact with you, keep him nearby so that you will notice the early signs of hunger, including:

- restlessness—while asleep or awake

- moving his head back and forth and wrinkling his brow

- putting his hand to his mouth

- making sucking motions and sounds

- licking his lips and sticking out his tongue

- making soft murmuring noises that grow louder

■ Don't wait until your baby cries to offer your breast. He is more likely to show an interest in breastfeeding if he is in a light sleep, slightly drowsy, or just barely awake. You can increase the likelihood of your baby learning to breastfeed by:

- keeping your baby near you during the day and at night. This will give your baby a chance to become familiar with your smell, to hear your heartbeat, and to find his way to your breast. In addition, sleeping near your baby at night makes it easy to take advantage of the increased nighttime production of prolactin.

- encouraging your baby to suck at your breast by using a nursing supplementer (see pp. 80–81).

- gradually moving your baby from bottle to breast. A good first step might be to offer a bottle of your expressed breastmilk or infant formula while your baby is held skin-to-skin in your arms. Some babies are more likely to attach to the breast if a bottle nipple or nipple shield is placed on the breast at the beginning of the feeding. Over time you will want to remove the nipple shield and place your baby directly on your breast.

- keeping a positive attitude. Depending on your baby's age, experience with artificial nipples, and personality, it may take many tries before he readily accepts your breast. It may help to know that mothers who wean their babies from the breast to the bottle often meet resistance as well. They expect that it will take time before their baby warms up to a new way of feeding. Weaning from the bottle to the breast is no different. Your baby's cool reaction to your breast may seem like a personal rejection, but he is simply telling you that this new way of feeding is unfamiliar.

Feeding Your Baby a Supplement

Whether you are relactating or inducing lactation, it is very common to have little or no milk when you start. Frequent suckling will stimulate milk production, but the quantity of milk produced may not be enough to satisfy your baby's need for food. Most mothers use infant formula to bridge this gap; others—especially those who are relactating because their babies cannot tolerate other foods—use donor human milk from a milk bank until their own milk supply is sufficient. Whatever you decide to use, it is important to make sure that your baby is adequately nourished during this period of rapid growth.

The nursing supplementer has the advantage of ensuring adequate nutrition while, at the same time, ensuring that the breasts are stimulated sufficiently to promote good milk production. As your milk supply increases, your baby will take less food from the supplementer. Offering your breast without the supplementer several times each day will help your baby more easily make the transition away from the supplementer when the time comes.

Some families supplement their babies at the breast using a syringe, and others choose cup feeding and simply offer the breast for comfort during this period. If a baby is regularly fed by bottle, he may not suck effectively at the breast. But some parents do use the bottle for some of their baby's feedings. It is important to keep breastfeedings and bottle-feedings in proportion. Recognize the bottle as a risk factor that may make breastfeeding more difficult. But don't be too critical of yourself if you find that using the bottle sometimes makes this period a little easier.

Getting Milk—When and How Much?

The timing and amount of milk production vary quite a bit. It can be anywhere from a few days to several weeks before you see any milk. Once milk is present, you may go on to produce all that your baby needs—or only a part of it. Women relactating for their homemade babies are at a biological advantage. If you have had a recent pregnancy and produced milk for a period of time afterwards, you may find that your milk supply rebuilds more quickly and more abundantly than the milk supplies of mothers who have never been pregnant or were pregnant some time ago.

Your milk supply very much depends on the "baby" and "brain" parts of the breastfeeding equation. The baby's stimulation of the breast and the signals the breast sends to the brain are central to all breastfeeding situations. But emotions and beliefs also play a role.

If the mother is under a lot of stress, adrenalin and other stress hormones are released. Adrenalin works like prolactin to stimulate milk production, but, unlike oxytocin, adrenalin inhibits milk release. Stress hormones were useful in earlier, more dangerous times when women often had to flee with their babies. They were unable to breastfeed while on the run, but once they found shelter plenty of milk was available. Avoiding very stressful situations if possible, and learning how to relax through them if they are unavoidable, are adaptive behaviors that can help ensure that milk is always available.

What a woman believes about her ability to breastfeed is also very important. We don't completely understand why, but experience suggests that women who are confident in their ability to produce milk—and are supported by their families, their health care providers, and members of their community—often lactate more easily and produce more milk than women who are uncertain of their ability to feed their babies at the breast or have little support. This, in part, explains why breastfeeding tends to be easier with second and subsequent children.

To some extent, you can create a breastfeeding-friendly environment by selecting health care providers who support your efforts, by enlisting the support of family and friends, and by involving yourself in a mother-to-mother breastfeeding support group such as La Leche League. You may not be able to eliminate all of your doubts about your ability to breast-feed, but creating a supportive environment will go a long way toward making relactation or induced lactation a good experience for you and your family.

Increasing Your Milk Supply/Reducing the Supplement

Once you start to produce even a small amount of milk, you will want to gradually reduce the amount of supplement you give to your baby. Keep in mind that every drop of mother's milk is nutritional and immunological gold, so that your baby will benefit even if you have only a small amount.

Your baby will continue to need the supplement—at least at first—to ensure that both his body and his brain continue to grow well and that he has the energy to suck eagerly at your breast. If he is gaining nicely (4–8 ounces a week or a pound or two a month) and breastfeeding at least eight times in each 24 hours, you can steadily reduce the amount of supplement while maintaining or even increasing the amount of time he spends breastfeeding.

Eliminating about 5–10 percent of your baby's formula intake at any one time is plenty. If your baby feeds eight times in 24 hours and each feeding is approximately 7 1/2 ounces, his total intake is 60 ounces. Therefore, you could safely eliminate 3–6 ounces of formula. You may want to spread this out over several feedings. For example, you might give your baby 1/2–1 ounce less in six of his feedings and leave the other ones as they are.

Many mothers who find that they produce more milk early in the day (due to higher prolactin levels at night) prefer to reduce the supplement more during that period. They decrease three morning feedings by 1–2 ounces each, for instance. Some mothers are able to give a couple of breastmilk-only feedings early in the day or during the night and add the supplement to the other feedings.

There is no right or wrong way to combine breastmilk and supplement feedings. What is most important is that you reduce the supplement slowly and check your baby's weight as well as the number of wet and dirty diapers frequently. No matter what your baby's primary source of food, you will want to see at least six heavy, wet diapers each day and one or more bowel movements, depending on your baby's age (see pp. 32–33).

If your baby goes through a sudden growth spurt, you may have to delay further cutbacks or even increase the supplement a little. This does not mean that you are producing less milk but only that your baby's needs have increased faster than your milk supply. With a little patience and careful attention to frequent sucking stimulation, you'll catch up and be able to eliminate more of the formula supplement.

This process may go quickly or it may take many weeks. Some mothers —especially those who are breastfeeding adopted babies—are able to eliminate the supplement entirely only after their babies are eating solid foods. For these mothers it is a long journey, but, with the introduction of solid foods at about 6 months of age, their breastfeeding experience more and more resembles that of mothers whose babies were born to them.

Galactagogues

From the earliest times, many cultures have singled out foods and herbs that "make" milk. Such foods and herbs are referred to as *galactagogues*.

There is little evidence that these foods and herbs actually cause an increase in milk production, but the belief that they work may be enough to convince the brain (pituitary gland) to make more milk. Early relactation clinics in Africa often asked mothers to drink milk (an unusual practice for adults in that region), promising them that it would make their milk flow like the river Nile. This practice was just one part of a comprehensive program of support that enabled these women to resume full lactation for their babies.

Many breastfeeding mothers in Europe firmly believe that special breastfeeding teas are the key to a good milk supply. Most of the ingredients have not been proven to have this effect, though, and some of them—most notably peppermint—are known to decrease milk production. Only a very few commonly used galactagogues have been studied. All of them act on the pituitary gland to increase prolactin production and stimulate milk production. Among those that appear to be useful are:

- fenugreek—an herb previously used by dairy farmers to increase milk production in cows

- chlorpromazine—an antipsychotic drug

- metoclopramide—an antinausea drug

- domperidone—an antinausea drug

Research data with respect to relactation and/or induced lactation are limited. At this time, domperidone and metoclopramide appear to be the most effective, but caution is advised. Metoclopramide used for even brief periods of time can cause depression, and, although there are few known side effects with domperidone, the Food and Drug Administration (FDA) has issued a warning regarding the use of domperidone in breastfeeding mothers. Domperidone has been used with mothers of premature babies to help them maintain and increase their milk production over long periods until their babies are able to suckle effectively at the breast. It is best to talk with your health care provider before taking any medication.

Some adoptive mothers have participated in a program that involves the use of estrogen, progesterone, and domperidone given before the baby arrives, with continued use of domperidone afterwards. Initial reports from mothers are enthusiastic, although the amount of milk produced is similar to the amount reported by mothers who have had no medical intervention. And mothers with good community and medical support have also been shown to produce as much milk—with or without short-term use of either chlorpromazine or metoclopramide.

At this time there is no best way to ensure that a mother who chooses to relactate or induce lactation will have abundant milk. Women who live in cultures that believe that anyone with breasts can breastfeed seem to be at a psychological advantage with both relactation and induced lactation. But there are many exceptions to this rule. For the mother who wants to get her baby (back) to the breast and has enough support from the people who count in her life, it is certainly worth making the effort and seeing where it leads.

Deciding Not to Breastfeed

You may decide for many reasons not to continue your efforts to relactate or induce lactation. Perhaps your baby has been very unhappy with attempts to get him to the breast, maybe the effort involved has made it hard for you to enjoy your baby, or you may not have the kind of support you need to continue. In your disappointment, you may worry that you have failed or let your baby down.

Nothing could be further from the truth. By attempting to relactate or induce lactation—especially in a culture where breastfeeding is not the norm—you have already demonstrated your strong commitment to your baby's well-being, both physical and psychological. And because you are so aware of your baby's needs you may clearly see that the delight you have in each other is taking second place to breastfeeding. Sometimes the best thing you can do for your relationship with your baby is to stop breastfeeding, to shift your focus from producing milk to parenting.

If your baby is content to be at the breast, but there is little or no milk, you can continue to breastfeed him with a supplementer or switch to bottle-feeding and continue to use the breast to calm or comfort him.

If your baby is unhappy at the breast, bottle-feeding may be your best choice. You can still include many of the things you learned from breastfeeding.

- Always bottle-feed your baby in your arms so that feeding continues to be a social experience and a chance for you and your baby to be close.

- Watch for your baby's hunger cues just as you would if you were breastfeeding. Give formula on request so that your baby learns to recognize—and act on—his body's signals that he is hungry or full. Never pressure him to drink the last drop in the bottle.

- Use a nipple that makes your baby open his mouth wide. This promotes the development of his facial muscles.

- Choose a nipple with a small hole so that each feeding takes 20–30 minutes. If your baby still wants to suck after that, continue holding him and give him a pacifier.

- Switch sides to promote the development of your baby's hand-eye coordination. This may take some practice because you, like most adults, probably have a favorite side.

- Your bottle-fed baby still needs skin-to-skin contact. Make sure he has a chance to touch you—on your face, your arms, even your breast—while he is feeding. Undress him a bit so you can stroke his arms and legs. A baby massage course might also be useful. Bathing together is another way of ensuring that your baby gets a sufficient dose of skin-to-skin contact each day.

- Keep your bottle-fed baby close to you by using a carrier during the day and sharing a bed—or at least a room—with him at night. Studies have shown that babies who are cared for in this way cry much less.

- Talk with someone you trust about your own disappointment and sadness that breastfeeding was not the experience you had hoped for. Letting out these feelings—and then letting them go—will benefit your relationship with your baby.

- Enjoy your baby, love him to pieces, and keep in mind that breastfeeding, however long it may last, is only one episode in the long story of your life together.

13 Breastfeeding a Baby with Jaundice

Jaundice is a condition in which the eyes and skin look yellow. Jaundice occurs when there is too much bilirubin in the blood. During pregnancy, babies need extra red blood cells to meet their oxygen needs. After birth, these red blood cells break down, and bilirubin is released into the blood. The liver filters the bilirubin from the blood and removes it from the body through the stools. A baby's liver does not function fully until days or weeks after birth, so it is hard for even full-term babies to remove the large amount of bilirubin that collects after birth.

Meconium is a black, tarry substance found in the lower bowel of newborns. Meconium contains on average 450 mg of bilirubin. Early passage of meconium keeps bilirubin from being reabsorbed into the blood and decreases the risk of jaundice. When rules or routines limit the frequency or the length of breastfeedings, babies have fewer stools, and the bilirubin level rises. High levels of bilirubin can destroy brain cells and cause lasting damage.

Jaundice occurs in 50–75 percent of full-term babies and 75 percent of premature babies. Because jaundice in the breastfed newborn is a common, complex, and poorly understood problem, treatment of the breastfed baby with jaundice often causes confusion and concern for parents. In addition to making the eyes and skin look yellow, jaundice also causes many babies to be very sleepy and to breastfeed poorly.

Physiologic jaundice. Physiologic jaundice usually occurs 3 days after birth and disappears within 10–12 days. Recent studies have found no difference in peak bilirubin levels in breastfed versus bottle-fed babies.

However, breastfeeding may cause bilirubin levels to remain elevated for longer periods of time.

Though many doctors question the need to treat breastfed babies who have physiologic jaundice, other doctors recommend water or formula supplementation, phototherapy, or stopping breastfeeding for a brief period of time. Discuss the choices carefully with your baby's doctor to avoid unnecessary confusion.

Phototherapy (light treatment) involves the use of a fluorescent or fiber optic light source. When a baby is exposed to the light source, his bilirubin level goes down. If an overhead light source is used, a small mask may be placed over your baby's eyes. If your baby is placed on top of the light source, no mask is needed. Phototherapy will increase your baby's fluid needs, so remember to breastfeed frequently, every 1–3 hours.

Babies with jaundice, especially those receiving phototherapy, may be sleepy, so you will need to work at waking them for feedings. (See "Wake a sleepy baby," p. 29.)

Pathologic jaundice. Pathologic jaundice is caused by blood incompatibility or liver disease. Different from physiologic jaundice, pathologic jaundice occurs within 24 hours after birth, and the bilirubin level often rises quickly. Prompt medical attention is necessary.

Breastmilk jaundice. The cause of breastmilk jaundice is unclear. There may be a substance in the milk of some women that makes it hard for their baby to remove bilirubin from the blood. Breastmilk jaundice appears 5–7 days after birth. The bilirubin level usually peaks around 10–14 days. The baby's bilirubin level can stay high for several weeks or months. If the bilirubin level keeps going up, your baby's doctor may suggest that you substitute donor milk or infant formula for two or more breastfeedings for 1 or 2 days. Or, in rare cases, you may need to interrupt breastfeeding for 24 hours and pump or hand express. Because each of these options interferes with exclusive breastfeeding, discuss them fully with your baby's doctor before you make a decision.

Breastfeeding jaundice. Breastmilk jaundice should not be confused with breastfeeding jaundice. Breastfeeding jaundice occurs when babies are not breastfed often enough and appears 3–5 days after birth.

Breastfeed your baby whenever he shows signs of hunger, every 1–3 hours during the day and every 2–3 hours at night, or at least eight times in each 24-hour period. Fewer feedings result in fewer stools and increase the risk of jaundice.

Sometimes it is easy to identify the cause of jaundice. Often a more thorough medical examination is necessary. Jaundice that occurs after your baby leaves the hospital should be reported to your baby's doctor right away.

Preventing Jaundice

- Breastfeed as soon as possible after birth. Colostrum is a natural laxative that causes bowel movements (stools). Early, frequent stools help to remove bilirubin from the body.

Table 5. Jaundice in the Newborn

TYPE AND FREQUENCY	SIGNS	STARTS
Physiologic Jaundice ■ Affects 50–75 percent of newborns	Eyes and skin look yellow	3 days after birth
Pathologic Jaundice ■ Is very rare	Eyes and skin look yellow Baby may be sleepy and feed poorly	Within 24 hours of birth
Breastmilk Jaundice ■ Affects 1–2 percent of breastfed newborns	Eyes and skin look yellow Baby is: ■ alert and active ■ breastfeeding at least eight times in each 24 hours ■ gaining weight appropriately ■ having at least four stools a day	5–7 days after birth
Breastfeeding Jaundice ■ Varies	Eyes and skin look yellow Baby is: ■ sleepy ■ breastfeeding fewer than eight times in each 24 hours ■ losing more than 5–7 percent of birth weight ■ having fewer than four stools a day	3–5 days after birth

■ Breastfeed at least eight times in each 24 hours. Frequent feedings result in frequent stools, which increase the removal of bilirubin and decrease the risk of jaundice. After day 1, expect at least three stools a day for the next 3 days and at least four stools a day for the next 4 weeks.

■ Breastfeed well on the first breast before offering the second breast. This will produce high-calorie, high-fat feedings, which in turn will increase the number of stools and decrease the bilirubin level and the risk of jaundice.

■ Avoid water or formula supplements. As long as you have a good supply of colostrum or breastmilk and your baby is breastfeeding at least eight times in each 24 hours and passing at least four stools a day, continued breastfeeding is all your baby needs.

LASTS	CAUSE(S)	TREATMENT
10–12 days	Breakdown of excess red blood cells Immature newborn liver	Breastfeed at least eight times in each 24 hours Check bilirubin level as needed
Bilirubin level rises quickly and continues to rise until medical treatment has begun	Blood incompatibility (ABO, Rh) Liver disease	Medical evaluation Breastfeed at least eight times in each 24 hours Phototherapy Blood transfusion
Bilirubin level usually peaks 10–14 days after birth but can remain elevated for several weeks or several months	Unknown; may be something in the mother's milk	Breastfeed at least eight times in each 24 hours Check bilirubin level regularly If bilirubin level continues to rise after 14 days: ■ Start phototherapy ■ Alternate breastfeeds and banked donor milk or formula feeds ■ Interrupt breastfeeding for 24 hours
Bilirubin level will continue to rise until the baby is adequately fed	Underfeeding—fewer than eight breastfeedings in each 24 hours Underfeeding—limiting the length of each feeding (mother-led feeding) Poor breastmilk production, release, and/or transfer Inadequate stooling	Breastfeed at least eight times in each 24 hours Breastfeed as long as the baby wishes (baby-led feeding) Confirm signs of milk production, milk release, and milk transfer Supplement if necessary with breastmilk or formula

14 Breastfeeding a Baby with a Family History of Allergic Disease

Parents who have a personal or family history of allergic disease such as asthma, hay fever, allergic rhinitis, chronic ear infections, or eczema should seriously consider breastfeeding their babies. This is particularly important if both parents suffer from allergic disease or have a previous child with allergic problems.

Breastfeeding for at least the first year of life can reduce the incidence of allergic symptoms (gas, diarrhea, vomiting, fussiness, and skin rashes) and the development of food sensitivity and upper respiratory infections in sensitive babies. Early introduction of foods other than human milk greatly increases the risk for food allergies. Human milk alone is recommended for the first 6 months. All formula and solid food supplements should be avoided.

When foods other than human milk are introduced, the new foods should be added one at a time at weekly intervals. This will let you clearly identify those foods that produce allergic symptoms.

Cow's milk, eggs, peanuts, peanut butter, and wheat should be avoided completely during the first year of life. After the first year, cow's milk and wheat can be added, but eggs should be avoided until 18 months of age and peanuts and peanut butter avoided until 3 years of age. This will not eliminate the development of sensitivity to these foods but will greatly reduce the likelihood of sensitivity. Our understanding of allergic disease is constantly changing. It is best to talk with your baby's doctor before you introduce any foods other than human milk.

If infant formula must be used, avoid formulas containing cow's milk and use formulas containing soy instead. For extremely sensitive babies—or if severe symptoms occur, and breastfeeding is not possible or human milk is not available—your baby's doctor can suggest a hypoallergenic formula (one that does not cause allergies).

Occasionally allergic symptoms develop in exclusively breastfed babies. Food proteins can be found in human milk in small quantities. For extremely sensitive babies, these proteins may occur in large enough amounts to cause allergic symptoms. In order to identify the cause of the symptoms, the mother's diet needs to be restricted.

Foods eaten by the mother that most often cause reactions in the baby are cow's milk, eggs, nuts, and wheat. You will need to eliminate these foods from your diet for 3 weeks, then re-introduce the foods one at a time, leaving 5–7 days between. It is unlikely that all the foods are the cause of the symptoms. By re-introducing the foods one at a time, it should be possible to determine which foods are the cause.

If the restricted diet does not improve your baby's symptoms, your diet can be returned to normal immediately, and your baby's doctor should be consulted. If your baby's symptoms are severe, a board-certified allergist should be consulted before the foods are re-introduced.

The following suggestions complement the use of human milk in achieving the goal of fewer symptoms in allergic children.

- Reduce dust and dust mite exposure in the home. Cover your mattresses with special dust mite preventive covers, limit the use of wall-to-wall carpeting throughout the house, and change furnace filters frequently.

- Avoid bringing furry and feathered animals into the home during the first 5 years of a child's life. It is much easier to refuse a pet than to get rid of a pet that has become part of the family. If a pet is already part of the family, early exposure may actually lower the risk of pet-related allergies. Talk with your doctor or your baby's doctor before you add or remove a pet.

- Keep infants and children in a smoke-free environment. This includes the homes of friends and relatives as well as automobiles. Early and chronic exposure to smoke is associated with an increased incidence of respiratory illnesses and early onset of asthma.

■ Avoid child care settings, nursery school environments, and church nurseries. Heavy and early exposure to viral infections can cause chronic diseases such as ear infections and infectious asthma. Early and frequent viral diseases can cause a significant increase in allergic antibodies. If child care outside the home is necessary, choose a setting with fewer children, to reduce the potential for problems.

Breastfeeding, environmental controls, animal avoidance, smoke avoidance, and dietary management do not prevent allergic disease. However, in many cases, they will delay the onset of symptoms for many years and limit the severity of symptoms when they do occur. This will allow your baby to mature and be better able to handle any symptoms that do develop.

Science has shown time and again that breastfed babies, both allergic and nonallergic, have fewer acute infections, have less risk of chronic disease, and respond better to immunizations. Human milk is truly the food of choice for every baby.

15 Breastfeeding After Breast Surgery

Some women who have had breast surgery are able to breastfeed fully (without needing to give formula supplements) while others are not. Your ability to breastfeed will depend upon the location of the surgical incision, the amount of breast tissue removed, and whether nerves, blood vessels, or milk ducts were damaged in the process. If the surgical incision was near the nipple and areola, damage is more likely to have occurred. As you think about your breastfeeding goals, it is important to remember that any amount of breastfeeding benefits you and your baby.

The most common surgical procedures are breast implant surgery (placement of breast implants), breast reduction surgery (removal of breast tissue), lumpectomy (removal of a breast lump), and mastectomy (removal of a breast).

Breast Implant Surgery

Breast implants are used to enlarge an existing breast or to form a new breast after one has been removed. Many women with breast implants breastfeed fully, although breastfeeding problems are more common in women with implants than in women without implants. Sometimes incisions are made around or near the areola for cosmetic reasons. These types of incisions are more likely to cause lasting damage to milk ducts, nerves, and blood vessels.

Since breastfeeding offers so many benefits, women with implants are encouraged to breastfeed. If you are concerned about the condition of your breast implants, talk with your doctor about a magnetic resonance imaging (MRI) exam. This exam can show whether breast implants are intact or leaking.

If you are planning to have breast implant surgery, let your doctor know beforehand that you would like to protect your ability to breast-feed as much as possible. Breast implants are usually filled with silicone gel or saline (salt water). Regardless of the type of breast implant used, complications often occur. Before you decide to have surgery, be aware that:

- Complications from breast implant surgery can include pain, infection, leakage, rupture, and capsular contraction.

- Breast implant surgery may affect your ability to breastfeed.

- Breast implants will make future breast examinations more difficult.

- Breast implants seldom last a lifetime. You will likely need more surgery to repair, replace, or remove the implants.

- Breast implant surgery and/or treatment of complications may not be covered by your health insurance.

Silicone Gel–Filled Breast Implants

Silicone gel–filled breast implants were first used in the early 1960s. More than 2 million women in the United States alone have received silicone gel implants. In 1992 silicone gel implants were taken off the market after several studies reported a possible link between silicone gel implants and autoimmune disease, a condition in which the body's immune system attacks the body itself. Since then, researchers have studied the effects of silicone gel implants on women and their breastfed children and have found no evidence of an increase in either breast cancer or autoimmune disease. Because of ongoing concerns about the safety of silicone gel implants, the Food and Drug Administration (FDA) determined that silicone gel implants should be used only in women participating in approved studies.

Saline-Filled Breast Implants

Saline implants are thought to be safe and effective and are approved by the FDA for use in all women.

Breast Reduction Surgery

If your breasts were very large, and you experienced physical or emotional pain due to their size, you may have chosen to have breast reduction surgery. When a large amount of breast tissue is removed, nipples and areolas are sometimes repositioned on the newly formed breasts. Milk ducts, nerves, and blood vessels are often damaged in the process. This damage can cause numbness in the breast and nipple which may or may not go away. This loss of feeling can affect your ability to breastfeed as well as your sexual response.

Women who have had breast reduction surgery often find that their milk production is limited. If you have had breast reduction surgery, you can still breastfeed, but you may need to supplement with donor human milk or infant formula if your baby gains too little weight. Let your baby's doctor know that you have had breast reduction surgery, and check your baby's weight frequently during the early months.

Lumpectomy

Removal of a breast lump seldom affects your ability to breastfeed unless the incision is on or near the nipple and areola. If a cancerous lump is found while you are breastfeeding, and radiation or chemotherapy is necessary, you may need to stop breastfeeding.

Mastectomy

Breast cancer occurs in women of all ages and is the most likely cause for breast removal. Breast cancer treatments include removal of the breast lump, removal of the entire breast, radiation therapy, and chemotherapy. If only a single breast is removed, you can breastfeed on the remaining breast.

Making a Decision

Talk with your doctor (surgeon) before you have any breast surgery. Carefully discuss the benefits as well as the concerns. While your doctor will do his or her best to protect your ability to breastfeed, you may find after surgery that you are unable to breastfeed fully and must use formula supplements. As you adjust your breastfeeding goals, it may help to remember that any amount of breastfeeding benefits you and your baby. So enjoy this time together.

16 Combining Breastfeeding and Working

Many mothers who work outside the home continue to breastfeed. It takes a little extra planning, but the benefits are worth it (see "Benefits of Breastfeeding," p. 1).

- Breastfeeding keeps a mother and baby close even when they are apart.

- Breastmilk keeps babies healthy (especially those in group child care centers).

- Mothers of healthy babies miss less work, lose less income, and worry less about sick babies.

- Breastfeeding saves money; mothers who breastfeed do not have to spend their earnings on large amounts of infant formula or foods to replace their breastmilk.

Many mothers do not realize how easy it is to combine breastfeeding and working, so they stop breastfeeding when they return to work. However, as the number of working mothers increases, employers are becoming more supportive of breastfeeding. In the past, few employers considered breastfeeding beneficial, but today many see how breastfeeding can help their business. Breastfeeding and working can be a win-win-win situation for mother, baby, and employer.

Key Points to Think About

As you plan how you will combine breastfeeding and working, here are some key points to think about:

- How do you plan to feed your baby when you return to work?

- How will you express your milk or feed your baby during working hours?

- How will you complete your work duties and take care of your breastfeeding needs?

- How will you combine work duties and household chores?

Start planning while you are pregnant

Let your employer know as soon as possible that you are pregnant. Use this time to learn about your company's maternity policies, benefits, and work options. Discuss these options with your employer; suggest new options if necessary

- How long is your maternity leave? Is it paid or unpaid? How much leave can you take without losing your job or position? Does your national, state, or local government have a family medical leave law? (Some laws provide up to 12 weeks of unpaid maternity leave.)

- How many hours per week will you be expected to work when you return?

- Does your company offer work options such as flex-time (adjusting when you start and stop each work day), job sharing (sharing a full-time job with another person), part-time work, compressed work week (fewer days with longer hours), or telecommuting (working from home)?

- Does company policy allow you to leave the work site during the day or have an infant at work part or full time?

- Does your company offer on-site child care? If not, is this an option the company might consider?

- Does your company have a policy on breastfeeding or breastmilk expression at the work site? Does your company provide breast pumps or breastfeeding rooms? Does your company give employees time and support to breastfeed or express milk during the work day? (This is very important.)

Decide when you will return to work

Once you know the policies of your company, you can think about your options. The longer you and your baby can be together, the more stable your milk supply will be. Also, the older your baby is when you return to work, the less you may need to pump during the work day. It is best to take off as much time as possible. Whether you return to work after 6 weeks, 6 months, or 6 years will depend on your own needs and circumstances. For many mothers the decision to return to work is not a choice but a necessity. Mothers with limited sources of income and no paid maternity leave have to return to paid work as soon as possible.

Decide how many hours a week you would like to work and when

Those mothers able to return to work part time at first will find it easier to work and breastfeed. A part-time schedule gives you a chance to rest and care for yourself and your baby, and makes the return to work easier. Some mothers who return to work full time right away are able to work flexible hours that allow extra time during the work day for expressing milk or breastfeeding. Others compress their work week, completing a full-time schedule in fewer than 5 days—for example, working a 40-hour week as four 10-hour days or three 13-hour days.

Decide where and when you can express or breastfeed during working hours

If you plan to return to work shortly after your baby is born and want to express or breastfeed at the work site, think about where and when this can happen. You won't know how long breastfeeding or expressing your milk will take until after your baby is born and you have had a chance to practice, but you can plan ahead. Look for places at the work site where you can express your milk or breastfeed, such as a private office, a health clinic, or a child care center. You may need to be creative as you look for space, privacy, and comfort.

If you plan to use a breast pump, find out if your employer provides a pump and supplies, or ask for these as a baby gift.

Decide who will take care of your baby during working hours

Choosing child care is an important task. While cost and convenience are necessary considerations, choosing someone you trust who understands and supports breastfeeding is very important. Child care options include taking your baby to work with you; leaving your baby with an individual, in either your home or their home; taking your baby to a child care center; or arranging work schedules so that one parent is always available to care for your baby.

If you plan to breastfeed your baby during working hours, you might want to choose an individual or child care center near your work place or arrange to have your baby brought to you for feedings.

When you are interviewing different child care providers, ask them about their policies concerning breastfed babies. Choose someone who understands and supports breastfeeding and who is licensed or certified (especially if you are considering a group child care center). Take plenty of time to interview possible providers and make at least one unscheduled visit. You need to know that your baby will get the care you want.

Choose a provider who:

- provides a safe, clean place for your baby

- encourages you to breastfeed on-site when you drop off or pick up your baby, as well as during the day

- has an adequate number of trained staff who have experience with infant care and will help meet your baby's special needs

- is near your work site, if you are able to leave work to feed your baby

- knows how to safely handle your expressed breastmilk and feed your baby

If you have a child care center at your work site, let your employer know how much you value this employee benefit. If you do not have on-site child care, get information from other companies who provide this service and share the information with your employer.

Get support from your employer, supervisor, and co-workers

Before you begin your maternity leave, discuss your ideas with your supervisor and co-workers. Encourage them to support your efforts to breastfeed after you return to work. See if you can get them to commit their support in writing. Some ideas for building and maintaining support with your employer include:

- Talking to other working, breastfeeding mothers about their situations at their work sites. If they have had positive experiences, see if their supervisors would be willing to discuss the arrangement(s) with your employer. Sometimes employers are more willing to follow where others have already shown success, rather than being the first to offer special services.

- Sharing research data or publications on how your breastfeeding can help their business. For instance, breastfed babies are typically sick fewer times, even when placed in group day care centers. Less sickness on your baby's part means less absence on your part, which means better productivity for the company. One study found that nonbreastfeeding mothers were absent from the work site three times more often (due to babies' illnesses) than breastfeeding mothers.

- Investigating ways to meet your job responsibilities while you are breastfeeding, so that your employer, supervisor, and co-workers will agree that you are doing your fair share of the work.

Take care of yourself and your baby during your maternity leave

Enjoy this precious time with your baby to the fullest. Breastfeed early and often. This will help your baby learn good breastfeeding practices and help you establish a good milk supply. Avoid pacifiers, bottles, or foods other than breastmilk for the first 4 weeks after birth. These can confuse your baby and decrease your milk supply.

Learn how to express and collect your breastmilk

If you plan to have your breastmilk given to your baby during the workday, you will need to learn to express and collect your milk.

You can practice hand expression as soon as your milk su~~~increases, 5–7 days after birth. You can also begin to use~~hand pump, a battery-operated pump, or an electric pum~~..~"Choosing a Breast Pump," p. 144). Practice early and often so that you will have time to learn this important skill before you return to work. Your first attempts at milk expression may produce only enough milk to cover the bottom of the collection container. Don't get discouraged. Much like successful breastfeeding, successful milk expression comes with practice (see "Expression and Collection of Human Milk," p. 139).

After you have expressed your milk, you can store it in just about any food storage container. There are even plastic bags made just for breastmilk. Use something that is not likely to break, tear, or tip over in the refrigerator or freezer.

If you are expressing early on, and your baby is breastfeeding well, freeze your milk for later use. Label it with the date it was expressed. Breastmilk can be stored in a cool room for up to 5 hours, in the refrigerator for up to 5 days, in the freezer section of a refrigerator/ freezer for up to 5 months, or in an upright or chest freezer for up to 1 year.

As your baby gets older and your return to work gets closer, store your milk in single servings. Of course, your baby may want a bit more or less than this amount on any given day. If your baby seems hungrier than usual, feel free to make up larger servings for your baby's child care provider, or send along extra servings. Remember to adjust serving size as your baby grows.

Estimate the size of a single serving during the first 3 months

[handwritten: ×7 = 17.5 oz per day]

During the first 3 months, babies eat about 2 1/2 ounces each day for every pound they weigh. For example, an 8-pound baby would eat 2 1/2 ounces x 8 pounds, or 20 ounces a day. Divide this amount by the number of feedings, and you can estimate the size of a single feeding. If this 8-pound baby breastfeeds 10 times a day, 20 ounces ÷ 10 feedings = 2 ounces per feeding.

Introduce a new feeding method and/or a breastmilk substitute

Once your baby is breastfeeding well, about 4 weeks after birth, you can introduce a new feeding method. If you do this too soon, you can confuse your baby. However, if your work schedule requires that you be away from your baby during feeding times, you need to know that he will accept food from something other than the breast and from someone other than you.

What to substitute

Depending on your baby's age and ability, you can use expressed breastmilk, infant formula, or solid food. Doctors recommend breastmilk alone for the first 6 months. If you cannot provide breastmilk, your baby's doctor can recommend an infant formula. After the first 6 months, solid foods can be slowly introduced, but breastmilk or infant formula should still be fed through the first year of life.

How to substitute

You can use a spoon, cup, medicine dropper, hollow-handled medicine spoon, or bottle—whichever you, your baby, and your child care provider prefer. Should you choose to place the substitute in a bottle, try different nipple shapes and sizes until you find one that your baby will accept. Let someone other than you offer the substitute—your baby expects meals from you to come from your breast, not a cup or a bottle! In fact, you may want to leave the room during the feeding since some babies refuse substitutes when the real thing is nearby. Your baby's father, grandmother, babysitter, brother, or sister may be more than happy to offer the feeding.

Some mothers and babies avoid substitutes by reverse-cycle breastfeeding. Reverse-cycle breastfeeding means letting your baby sleep during the day while you are at work and breastfeeding in the evening and at night when you are together.

Decide how you will combine household chores and work duties

When both parents work full time outside the home, household chores are often shared. While cooking, cleaning, doing laundry, paying bills, grocery shopping, and running errands take time and energy, now breastfeeding and child care must be added to the to-do list!

■ Sit down with your partner and make a list of all your household chores.

■ Decide which chores can be put off, and divide up the rest.

Return to work

During your pregnancy and maternity leave, you laid out your plans. You and your baby have learned to breastfeed. Now it is time to put these plans into action (Figure 33).

2 weeks before your scheduled return to work

■ Discuss your plans with your supervisor. Assure her/him that you will be able to maintain your agreed-upon daily and weekly work schedule.

■ See how much time you will need each workday to wake, dress, feed yourself and your baby, and travel to child care and work.

■ Let your babysitter and baby spend time together so they can get to know one another.

■ Begin to establish a milk expression schedule, if you will be expressing milk at work.

■ If you will not be able to express milk at work, drop one feeding during the day and introduce a substitute so that your milk supply has a chance to adjust. If you need to drop a second daily feeding, wait 3–5 days.

■ Introduce a substitute to your baby at the time you would otherwise breastfeed.

■ Start making extra meals for you and your partner and storing them in the freezer.

1 week before your scheduled return to work

■ Continue your expression and breastfeeding schedule so that it will be close to what you will be doing when you return to work.

- Leave your baby with the babysitter for a few hours two or three times this week so they can get to know one another.

- Hold a dress rehearsal of your new morning routine on 1 or 2 days this week and make changes as needed.

- Try to get plenty of sleep so that you are ready for your return to work.

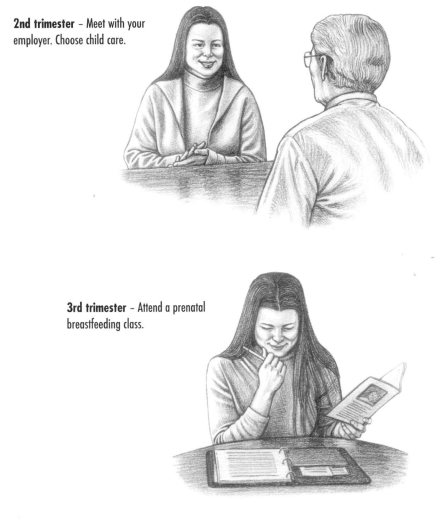

2nd trimester – Meet with your employer. Choose child care.

3rd trimester – Attend a prenatal breastfeeding class.

Figure 33
Many mothers combine breastfeeding and working. You simply need to plan ahead.

When you return to work

- If you return to work full time, work only 2 or 3 days the first week. For example, if your work week is Monday through Friday, return to work on a Wednesday or Thursday.

- Take one day at a time. If work has piled up while you were away, relax and do your best to catch up.

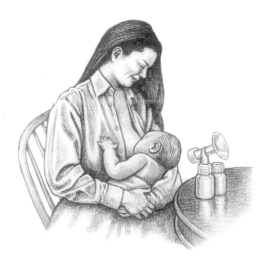

Birth - Breastfeed as soon as possible.

1–2 weeks - Breastfeed 8-12 times each 24 hours or every 1-3 hours.

2–4 weeks - Learn to express and collect your milk; freeze milk for later use.

4–10 weeks - Introduce a bottle or cup.

6–12 weeks - Delay your return to work for 12 weeks if possible.

2 weeks before you return to work - Decide how much time you will need each work day to get you and your baby ready.

1 week before you return to work - Hold a dress rehearsal.

After you return to work - Make the most of your time together.

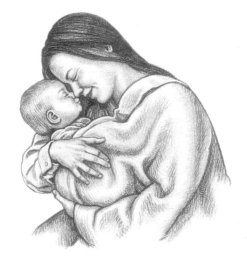

6am?

- Breastfeed your baby right before you leave him with the sitter. This will limit the amount of milk you will need to express while you are apart.

- Express or breastfeed according to your established routine. You will probably need to make small adjustments depending on your work schedule. Try to pump or breastfeed a little early rather than a little late. Many times the hours rush by and you may find yourself having gone longer than planned. Unfortunately, if you do not express or breastfeed, milk is more likely to leak from your breasts, you will be uncomfortably full, and your milk supply may decrease.

6pm

- Breastfeed your baby right after you return from work. If your breasts are very full or you have a long commute home, you may want to breastfeed before you leave the child care center. This will keep you and your baby happy. Ask your child care provider not to feed your baby for 1–2 hours before your planned return, so that he will be ready to eat when you get there.

- Breastfeed more often in the evenings and on weekends when you and your baby are together. This will help to maintain your milk supply.

- Talk to your supervisor about how things are going. Be positive and thankful, but also be open and honest if there are difficulties.

- Take care of yourself. Commit to getting enough sleep and eating a healthy diet.

- Give your baby at least one substitute feeding each day during any days off work (weekends, vacations, holidays).

Regardless of how well you prepare for your return to work, there will still be a period of adjustment. Excitement, nervousness, guilt, sadness, and joy are a few of the emotions you may experience. These feelings are normal. With time you will adjust priorities and establish routines, and your confidence in your decision will grow. Support and encouragement from people around you are important, so don't hesitate to ask for help.

Any amount of breastfeeding is wonderful. More important than how long you breastfeed or how often is that it be enjoyable for mother and baby.

17 Breastfeeding Beyond the First Year

Breastfeeding isn't just for babies!

Many mothers and toddlers cherish the special relationship that breast-feeding provides and continue to breastfeed beyond the first year. Most health professional organizations recommend that children be breastfed for 2 years or more. Depending on the needs of your child, you can continue to breastfeed for 2, 3, or more years. Breastfeeding an older baby or toddler can be rewarding as well as challenging.

Are there benefits to breastfeeding beyond the first year?

The benefits of breastfeeding continue as long as you continue to breastfeed. Although the emotional benefits of breastfeeding are most often given as the reason for breastfeeding an older baby or toddler, breastfed babies of all ages enjoy better health. Other foods provide toddlers with important nutrients, but only breastmilk contains anti-bodies that play a role in preventing disease.

- Breastmilk can provide toddlers with up to a third of their calorie, protein, and calcium needs.

- Breastmilk continues to be a source of antibodies that fight infection and illness during the second year and beyond.

- If a breastfed toddler does get sick, the illness often lasts for a shorter period of time.

- If a sick toddler refuses to eat, breastmilk may be the only source of nourishment that he will accept.

- Studies suggest that breastfeeding for a longer period of time may result in even smarter babies.

Mothers also benefit from breastfeeding beyond the first year.

- Women who breastfeed exclusively for the first 6 months are less likely to get pregnant, so child spacing is easier.

- The longer a mother breastfeeds, the less risk she has of breast, ovarian, and uterine cancer.

- Women with diabetes find that their insulin needs continue to be lower while they are breastfeeding.

- Breastfeeding makes weight loss easier for many mothers.

For older babies who prefer to "eat and run," breastfeeding offers a quick snack. Breastfeeding also provides help in falling asleep, comfort after getting hurt, and reassurance when mothers and babies are reunited after a separation. Because breastfeeding is something that only mothers can do for their babies, many busy mothers, especially those returning to work or school, find that breastfeeding makes it easier for them to reconnect with their babies at the end of the day.

Years later, a mother who breastfed her toddler can still recall his tiny hands gently patting or rubbing her face during breastfeeding. She remembers the special love she felt as her baby looked into her eyes and smiled, still attached to her breast. She can also recall the sweet baby sounds and simple words that told her how special breastfeeding was to her baby.

Is breastfeeding a toddler different from breastfeeding an infant?

Breastfeeding a toddler is very different from breastfeeding an infant. Most breastfeedings are short and sweet, but the frequency can vary from once every other day to several times each day. Because toddlers eat a wide variety of foods, they don't need to breastfeed at certain times. If a mother and baby are out and about during the usual feeding time, the older baby will usually accept some other food or drink without a fuss. Some toddlers will insist on breastfeeding, regardless of the time and place. As they get older, they will be more willing to wait.

Breastfeeding an older baby can be an adventure. Toddlers are very aware of what's going on around them. Don't be surprised if your toddler lets go of the breast to watch the cat, smile at dad, or simply react to a noise. You might think this means that your baby is losing interest in breastfeeding. However, this behavior is normal and is one of the ways babies learn. Some toddlers turn away from the breast but don't let go, testing the ability of the breast to stretch! This doesn't mean that breastfeeding must stop. But because some toddlers are so easily distracted, you may need to breastfeed in a quiet place.

As babies get older, sleep patterns change, too. Some breastfed babies sleep for long periods of time right from the start, and by 1 or 2 years of age are sleeping all night. Other older babies continue to wake at night to breastfeed, especially if they are not offered regular meals and snacks during the day. Parents' habits also affect the older baby's sleeping schedule. If you are a night owl, your toddler may be one also.

What will my friends and family think?

Everyone has opinions about how you should raise your baby. And, unfortunately, most are eager to share their opinions, which often include feelings about how long you should breastfeed. You and your partner will have to decide what is best for you and your baby and ignore advice that is not supportive.

Family members may frown on long-term breastfeeding. They may believe that breastmilk provides no nutrition or benefits after the first year. The whole idea of breastfeeding a baby that looks like a child may make them feel uncomfortable. And they may make it their mission to convince you to change your mind about continuing to breastfeed.

Be prepared to deal with family members' questions and comments. Share the facts about breastfeeding to win their support when possible. If you are asked repeatedly to say how long you intend to breastfeed, you can truthfully say that you have started weaning. Weaning actually does begin when your baby starts to eat foods other than breastmilk. However, the end of breastfeeding may not happen for many months or years.

Many people believe that breastfeeding beyond a certain age will make children too dependent or "tied" to mom. But research suggests that just the opposite is true. Children who form a secure attachment with their mother are better able to form relationships with others and are more likely to be independent.

Negative comments from family and friends are seldom meant to be hurtful. Your family and friends care about you and your child and want what is best for you, even if their information is wrong. Find out their specific concerns so that you will know how to respond. Tell them what the doctor or other expert has said about breastfeeding an older child. Overall, most parents find that their family and friends quickly get used to the idea of breastfeeding an older baby. Many women who breastfed a year or more say that at first they couldn't picture themselves breastfeeding a toddler. But over time, breastfeeding a walking, talking toddler began to feel natural and normal.

What challenges will I face breastfeeding an older baby?

Breastfeeding in Public

Many mothers continue to breastfeed beyond the first year but do so only in a private place or in their home. In some cultures, breasts may be seen as sexual objects rather than body organs designed to nourish babies. Most people accept the need to breastfeed a young infant whenever and wherever he gets hungry. They usually smile with approval or just look away. However, they don't feel the same about older babies breastfeeding. A common belief is that a mother who breastfeeds an older baby is doing so for her own satisfaction. Some mothers have experienced rude comments or staring, or have been asked to leave a place. For some people, seeing an older baby breastfeeding stirs up feelings of anger or disgust.

There are many ways to handle questions, comments, or looks that may make you feel uncomfortable. First, draw as little attention as possible by covering up with a shawl, scarf, or child's blanket. Second, ask a family member or friend to hold your baby or toddler so that he doesn't ask to breastfeed in public by pulling at your blouse or breast. Third, teach your toddler to use a code word for breastfeeding that does not suggest that you may still be breastfeeding. Most toddlers will ask to breastfeed even if the mother has never done so in public.

Toddlers can wait to breastfeed and can eat other foods, so you may find it easier to just avoid breastfeeding in public.

Many countries have laws that protect a mother's right to breastfeed in public. As breastfeeding becomes more common, women will care most about the needs of their children and least about the opinions of others.

Teeth and Biting

Many mothers worry about what will happen when their baby gets teeth. Babies often have six to eight teeth by 1 year of age and biting issues already have passed. It may be comforting to know that it's not possible for your baby to breastfeed and bite at the same time. When a baby is latched on well, the mother's nipple extends far back into the baby's mouth. The nipple does not come into contact with the baby's teeth. Not all babies bite, and biting does not have to end breastfeeding.

You can reduce the chances that your baby will bite. Biting tends to occur near the end of a feeding when a baby is full or when a baby really isn't hungry. Watch for signs that your baby has finished feeding and remove him from the breast. Biting may also occur while a mother is talking on the phone or not interacting with her baby. Give your baby your full attention while breastfeeding, and breastfeed in a quiet place.

Sometimes biting issues begin early if a baby is allowed to bite or pinch a mother's arm, neck, or face during play. A baby does not know that biting the breast is different, so do not allow playful biting involving yourself or anyone else. Babies find comfort in rubbing their gums against something when their gums are sore during teething. Try rubbing your baby's gums with your fingers and use a chilled, firm teething ring to soothe his gums between breastfeedings.

If your baby does bite, avoid smiling, laughing, or reacting in a way that makes your baby think it was funny or cute. Calmly push your baby's face into your breast. This causes the baby to release the nipple. Then remove your baby from the breast and firmly say "no." Toddlers are able to understand your dislike for their behavior. Wait until the next usual feeding time to allow your baby to breastfeed again. Biting may occur only once if dealt with quickly. Like other stages in your baby's life, biting will become a thing of the past.

Will breastfeeding cause my toddler not to eat or grow well?

Breastfeeding toddlers will usually eat solid foods with a variety of flavors and textures if the foods are introduced between 6 and 12 months of age. That seems to be the time when babies are ready to learn to eat and enjoy solid foods. Regular meals and snacks plus continued breast-feeding will help to keep your older baby healthy.

Some parents put off adding foods because they think foods are not needed until after 1 year of age if the baby is breastfeeding. When parents delay giving foods at the age when babies are ready, eating may become a battle. As a result, the toddler may not grow as well as expected. Toddlers who refuse to eat or who eat very little have usually been allowed to breastfeed too frequently in place of eating solid foods.

Parents may put off adding chunky or table foods until after 1 year because they are worried about choking. While it is a good idea to avoid some foods like hot dogs, grapes, or nuts, most soft foods are safe for toddlers. If toddlers have been offered only smooth or pureed foods, they may fear foods with texture and refuse to eat. But if foods with texture and shape are added gradually, the baby will learn to handle the foods without a problem.

Where can I find support in my community for breastfeeding an older child?

Mothers who are breastfeeding toddlers often find strength in numbers. Many communities offer mother-to-mother support groups sponsored by La Leche League International. La Leche League usually offers organized meetings as well as telephone counseling. (See "Where Can I Find Help?" p. 175.)

Regardless of how long you and your baby decide to breastfeed, be confident in knowing that you have given your baby the very best.

18 Especially for Teens

"Are you going to breastfeed?"

Chances are you have heard this question many times during your pregnancy. And you have probably discovered that some people have strong feelings about breastfeeding and are eager to share those feelings, both good and bad. Perhaps your family and friends have already told you the "facts" about breastfeeding.

Family and friends can be a good source of information. But if your family or friends did not breastfeed or found that breastfeeding was hard, you may want to ask your health care provider to introduce you to a mom who has breastfed or, better yet, who is breastfeeding now. An experienced mom knows firsthand the challenges that you will face as you try to balance school, work, friends, family, and motherhood!

"Are my breasts too big or too small?"

"Will breastfeeding be painful?"

"How can breastfeed after I go back to school?"

"Do I have to eat only healthy foods?"

"Can I smoke or drink alcohol if I breastfeed?"

"What if my boyfriend doesn't want me to breastfeed?"

"Can I use birth control?"

The answers to these questions and more are found in this book and in the following stories from other teen moms. These are real stories from real moms.* And, just like you, they want to be the best mother that they can be.

Why should I breastfeed?

Breastfeeding is good for you and your baby!

Breastfed babies are smarter. Babies who breastfeed have better brain development, do better on IQ tests, and usually do better in school.

Breastfed babies have fewer ear infections, less constipation and diarrhea, and less risk of asthma, allergy, and childhood obesity. Breastfeeding, putting your baby on his back to sleep, and keeping your baby away from second-hand smoke all reduce the risk of sudden infant death syndrome (SIDS). (See pp. 36–37 for suggestions on how to keep your baby safe from SIDS.)

Breastfeeding protects you, too. Mothers who breastfeed usually lose weight easier and have less bleeding after childbirth. They also have less risk of breast, ovarian, and uterine cancer. This may not seem important now, but it can be important as you get older.

What other teens say about why you should breastfeed

"I believe, right now you are trying to decide if you should breastfeed or not. Just try it. If you find that you have problems, do not give up real quick. Call someone you know who has breastfed. Tell them you are having a problem. Talk it over with someone you trust. Clear your mind of all the advice, and all the wrong ideas you have been given about breastfeeding. Start fresh. Know that it is best for your baby to breastfeed and that you are going to do it." —*Kayla*

"Breastfed babies are less likely to get sick with stomach problems, ear infections, and colds. Breastfeeding keeps your baby healthy. Healthy babies are easier to take care of. It is easier for the mother and baby to breastfeed." —*Latisha*

---

* I am most grateful to the people at Best Start Social Marketing for their kindness in allowing me to share these stories with you. The names of the mothers have been changed to protect their privacy.

"It is easier to breastfeed. I don't have to make a bottle, and worry about boiling it or having the nipples ready. Breastmilk is right there. It's always there. The milk doesn't spoil. It is so easy, simple, and fast and it is so good for the baby. It is the best thing for me and my baby. That's what I went with." —*Hannah*

"Breastfeeding allows you to hold your baby in your arms and look into its eyes. This lets you feel all the love in the world. The way your baby looks at you will just melt your heart." —*Jasmine*

Is it hard to breastfeed?

Some people think that because breastfeeding is "natural" it must be easy. While making milk is natural, breastfeeding is a skill that you and your baby must learn. Learning to breastfeed takes practice and patience. But once you learn, breastfeeding is easy.

What other teens say about learning to breastfeed

"When I started breastfeeding I was real excited. But my baby did not want to take the breast at first. He rejected it a lot. The nurse said to be patient and he will do it. Then he breastfed fine." —*Tamika*

How does breastfeeding make you feel?

Breastfeeding is the one thing that you can do for your baby that no one else can do. It is a good way to let family and friends know that you are this baby's mother and that the two of you have a special relationship. Mothers who breastfeed have a special bond with their babies and are more confident in their ability to care for their babies.

What other teens say about how it feels to breastfeed

"It gives me a proud feeling to breastfeed. An older woman walked up to me. She said, 'You know, I'm really proud of you because today you don't see young parents wanting to breastfeed their baby. They want to throw a bottle in their mouth and run out the door. But you are doing good.' She made me feel good." —*Emma*

"It makes me feel proud to breastfeed. I am giving my daughter something no one else can give her. I help her survive. It makes me feel really good." —*Shantell*

"I feel proud that I breastfeed. Many people said that I am too young to breastfeed. You are never too young. I mean, if you have a baby, you are not too young to breastfeed." —*Lee*

"I like to breastfeed because I feel more mature. I feel like I am an adult because I have always been thought of as a child. Once I started breastfeeding, people stopped treating me like a child. It makes me feel more mature to breastfeed." —*Niesha*

"I think it is just a general feeling that I get, because I know I'm giving something back to my baby. I watch her grow. It is really neat. I sit and think she is getting this from me. It is a great feeling." —*Grace*

"Most people think that teens should not get pregnant. Well I did. It might have been a mistake. It might have been on purpose. But, at least I am being careful to make sure my baby grows up healthy by breast-feeding." —*Ava*

How do I know if my baby is getting enough to eat?

Just remember—nothing comes out the bottom unless something goes in the top! As long as your baby has lots of poopy and wet diapers and is gaining the right amount of weight, you can be sure he is getting enough to eat. If you are worried about your milk supply, talk with your baby's health care provider.

What other teens say about babies getting enough to eat

"That's why I like to breastfeed. I don't have to worry if my baby is getting enough to eat. I can breastfeed for as long as she wants to. As long as my baby has at least six wet diapers and four bowel movements a day, then I know she is getting enough breastmilk." —*Brianna*

How will I survive with no sleep?

Breastfeeding saves time and energy, especially at night. There is no formula to mix, measure, and warm, so nighttime feedings are easier. Many mothers lie down to breastfeed at night so they can rest while their baby is feeding. Talk with your baby's health care provider about how to do this easily and safely.

What other teens say about nighttime feedings

"I decided to breastfeed so my baby would be healthy. Also, I don't have to carry bottles when I go places. I don't have to get up during the night to make bottles." —*Jada*

Doesn't breastfeeding tie you down?

Caring for a baby takes time, no matter how he is fed. Life is never simple, especially for busy teens, but breastfeeding can make life easier. Mothers who breastfeed usually have one hand free to eat a meal, catch up on homework, or talk on the telephone. Breasts and babies are portable, so mothers who breastfeed find it easier to come and go.

What other teens say about the time spent breastfeeding their babies

"It doesn't tie you down to breastfeed. It gives you more time with your baby. When you bottle-feed anyone can feed your baby. But when you breastfeed you have to spend time with your baby. So it gives you extra time to be with your baby and to bond with your baby." —*Zoe*

"I think it makes the baby feel safe and secure to breastfeed and become more attached to me. My baby knows that I am his momma. It is not like my baby is going to be so hung up on me that I can't do anything." *Claire*

Can I breastfeed if I have to go back to school?

Many teens (and even older mothers!) continue to breastfeed after they go back to school. It just takes a little extra planning. Be sure to read "Combining Breastfeeding and Working," p. 112, since a lot of the information applies to mothers returning to school as well.

- Let your teachers know that you plan to continue breastfeeding and that, since breastfed babies are healthier, mothers who breastfeed miss fewer days of school.

- Decide who will take care of your baby while you are away.

- If your child care provider is near the school, see if you can leave school to breastfeed during school hours.

- If you are unable to breastfeed during the day, your baby can be fed your expressed (pumped) milk or infant formula.

- If you plan to have expressed milk fed to your baby, you will need to learn to express and store your milk (see "Expression and Collection of Human Milk," p. 139).

- Ask your teachers or the school nurse to suggest a private place where you can express milk during school hours.

What other teens say about going back to school and continuing to breastfeed

"Don't worry about having to go to school because you can still breast-feed in between. If you're just going to breastfeed at night, that's better than not breastfeeding at all." —*Faith*

What if my baby's father doesn't want me to breastfeed?

Talk with your baby's father about the benefits of breastfeeding for you and your baby. Encourage him to talk with other guys whose girl-friends or wives have breastfed. Help him separate breastfeeding facts from myths. Let him know how much you need his support as you learn to be a mother to your baby, and help him spend time with his baby, too.

What other teens say about how their boyfriend or husband feels about breastfeeding

"After our baby was born, my boyfriend complained a lot when I breastfed our baby. It was like he had no part in it. He would go sit somewhere else, because I was not paying any attention to him. I told him to sit with me while I breastfed. This made him feel like he was more involved. Soon he got used to having me breastfeed. Now it's like a family thing." —*Rebecca*

"You can pump your milk and have your boyfriend feed the baby, so he can also have that special bond with the baby." —*Victoria*

"My husband wanted me to breastfeed, not just for the cost of it but for health and he likes to watch me do it." —*Madeline*

"When it is time to put the baby to sleep, the father can do that. Then he can have his own special time with the baby." —*Sophia*

What teen dads say about breastfeeding

"Besides the bonding, it is much cheaper to breastfeed. It's just the natural thing to do." —*Dwight*

"There is a real bond between the mother and child when they breast-feed. I see that bond between the two of them. Every mother should feel that bond." —*Dylan*

Can I use birth control?

If you are having sex but do not want to get pregnant, make sure you use birth control. Talk with your partner and your health care provider about the type of birth control that is best for you.

Nonhormonal methods include a diaphragm, sponge, intrauterine device (IUD), condom, and spermicidal cream, foam, or jelly. Hormonal methods include the pill, patch, shot, and ring. Hormonal methods that contain only progesterone are thought to be safe. Hormonal methods that contain estrogen can limit milk production.

If you decide to use a hormonal method, wait until your milk supply is well established (about 6 weeks after your baby's birth) to be safe, and use a method that contains only progesterone. You may want to stay away from the shot and use the pill, patch, or ring, which can be stopped easily if your milk supply goes down.

What other teens say about birth control

"If teens were taught ways to talk about sex with their partners before it happens, they'd make better decisions, either not having sex or having safer sex." —*Acacia*

"Teens should also learn about contraception even if they *don't* plan on having sex. Be prepared, because you never know when something could change your mind ... or your life." —*Ashanti*

"Teens need to respect themselves and not be afraid to refuse sex without a condom or go to a clinic to get birth control." —*Melissa*

What teen dads say about birth control

"Since Laretha had the baby, we talk about birth control. I think the safest type of birth control for us at this time is to use the condom and the sponge. But whatever she chooses, I will support her." —*Joseph*

"There are so many methods of birth control. It is always best to discuss the best type of birth control method with a doctor." —*Anthony*

Can I breastfeed in public?

You can breastfeed wherever you feel comfortable. Some mothers are shy at first about breastfeeding in front of family or friends. But with a little practice, you can learn to breastfeed without your breasts showing (Figure 34). Some new mothers like to practice in front of a mirror so they can see which tops work best for breastfeeding in public. If you are uncomfortable breastfeeding in public, you can always breastfeed at home.

Figure 34
With a little practice, you can learn to breastfeed without your breasts showing.

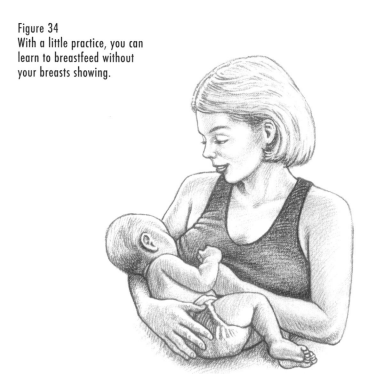

What other teens say about breastfeeding in public

"There are no rules to breastfeeding. You can breastfeed wherever you feel comfortable. Don't worry about what other people think. Your baby needs to eat like everyone else. You should be able to feed your baby where you want to." —*Maggie*

"For women who decide to breastfeed, do not let anyone tell you not to." —*Deanna*

"Before I go into the store, I feed him in the car after we stop in the parking lot. Then he is real calm and quiet in the store. It's just better for me. But in a restaurant, I'll breastfeed him while our food is being prepared. By the time our food is ready, he is nice and quiet, so I can eat." —*Kaitlyn*

"You can go anywhere wherever you want you can go. I just put a blanket over me and my baby. Just cover up. I don't really care what people think. Breastfeeding is right for my baby and right for me." —*Caroline*

Can I breastfeed if I have small breasts?

Breasts come in all shapes and sizes. Breast size and shape do not affect your ability to make milk. But nipple size and shape can sometimes make breastfeeding easier or harder. (See Figure 11, p. 18.) Be patient. With a little practice, your baby will learn to breastfeed on your breast.

What other teens say about breast size and shape

"When you have a baby, the milk is there. If your breasts are small, you still have enough milk. It doesn't make any difference. Your chest could be the smallest in the world and your body will still make enough milk." —*Geleen*

Do I have to eat only healthy foods?

While a healthy diet is best, mothers who eat "junk" food still produce enough milk to meet their baby's needs. Even if you like to eat "junk" food, try to also eat a variety of healthy foods each day, and drink enough so that you don't feel thirsty. All mothers make healthy milk. There are only a few medicines you cannot take when you are breastfeeding. Before you take any medicine, even those sold over the counter (without a prescription), talk with your baby's health care provider to make sure that what you are taking is okay.

What other teens say about eating while breastfeeding

"I think it has been exaggerated that if you don't eat the right things you won't have enough milk. I try to eat good food, but there are times when I just can't fix a home-cooked meal. I have always had enough milk for my baby. Remember that what you eat and drink can be passed through your breastmilk to your baby. Do not drink a lot of alcohol and do not take any medicines without talking to your doctor first." —*Diedre*

"Your body will change naturally to make you hungrier and thirstier. This will help you eat enough to meet the extra needs required for milk production. Generally, if you're eating enough to feel full, your milk will have everything your baby needs for normal growth and development." —*Yvonne*

"Very few people eat the right food all of the time. Eating junk foods and fast foods won't ruin your milk. Just remember that a variety of foods are needed for good health. Try to eat a balanced diet as often as possible." —*Maria*

What should I remember most?

Take one day at a time! Remember that taking care of a new baby is hard work, so feel good about the job that you are doing. Any amount of breastfeeding is good for you and your baby.

What other teens say is most important

"That the breast is beautiful. It was placed on your body for a reason, not just for some man to hang on. Think about the way you feel. If it is right for you to breastfeed, then do it. And if it's not, there are other choices, but try to breastfeed first." —*Isabella*

"Do not give up, if at first it doesn't seem to be going too well. It takes time to breastfeed. Even if you only breastfeed for a few weeks, you will still have a beautiful experience to share with others." —*Tara*

Just like you, all of these young mothers and fathers are trying hard to give their babies the best start in life. They hope that after hearing their stories, perhaps you will decide to breastfeed your baby, too!

19 Expression and Collection of Human Milk

Milk expression, like breastfeeding, is a learned art. It takes patience and practice. You do not need to express on a set schedule—simply watch your breasts, not the clock! Express whenever your breasts feel full or whenever it is convenient.

How often you express will depend upon your needs and the needs of your baby. For example, if you or your baby is unable to breastfeed for health reasons, you may need to express throughout the day and at night. If you need to be away from your baby for a period of time each day, you may need to express one or more times a day. But if you and your baby are seldom apart, you may need to express only once or twice a week.

If you have a good supply of milk, your breasts will tell you when you need to express. But if your milk supply is low, you may need to express more often to increase your supply.

Breastmilk can be collected by hand expression, hand pump, battery-operated pump, or electric pump. Mothers who plan to pump now and then will find that hand expression, a hand pump, a battery-operated pump, or a semi-automatic electric pump works well.

Mothers who need to pump daily or for many weeks or months may want to rent or purchase a fully automatic electric pump.

Even if you choose to use a breast pump, you should still learn to hand express, just in case your pump is not available. Hand expression is inexpensive and easy.

Your first tries at expressing your milk may produce only enough milk to cover the bottom of the collection container. Don't get discouraged.

It may take several days or weeks before you see an increase in the amount of milk obtained.

In the beginning you may want to express and collect from one breast while your baby breastfeeds from the opposite breast (Figure 35). Infant suckling will stimulate a let-down reflex and increase the flow of milk. As your confidence grows, you may want to express milk early in the morning or between feedings when your breasts seem full. It is important that you relax and think about your baby. This will encourage milk release and increase the amount of milk obtained.

Figure 35
Pumping one breast while your baby breastfeeds on the opposite breast can increase the amount of milk expressed.

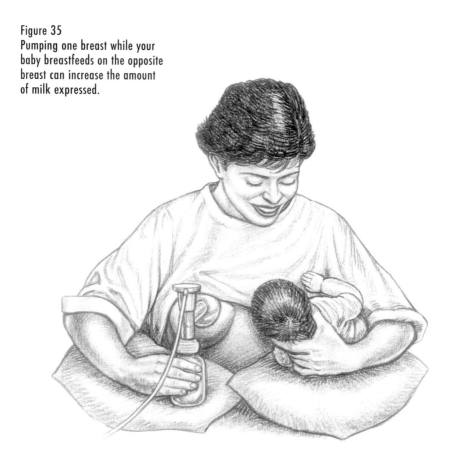

Hand Expressing

- Choose a quiet, comfortable place where you will not be disturbed. If necessary take the phone off the hook and lock the door.

- Get organized and gather all of your supplies together. Include a healthy snack and drink for yourself.

- Use a container with a wide opening. A mayonnaise or peanut butter jar works best. Wash the container in hot, soapy water and rinse well or clean it in a dishwasher.

- Wash your hands with soap and water and rinse well.

- Put warm water on your breasts. Taking a warm shower or tub bath, using warm washcloths, or soaking the breasts in a pan of warm water works well.

- Gently massage the breasts in a circular pattern using the flat part of your fingers (Figure 22, p. 54).

- Roll your nipple between your thumb and finger. This can cause a let-down reflex and make milk expression easier.

- Relax and think about your baby. This can help milk release and increase the amount of milk obtained. Looking at a picture of your baby, holding something he has worn, listening to music, or listening to a relaxation tape may also be helpful. Plan to do some relaxation exercises at least once a day even if you cannot do them just before pumping.

- Gently support the breast with one or both hands.

- Place your thumb and first two fingers opposite each other on your breast, about 1–2 inches from the base of the nipple.

- Press in toward your chest, then slowly bring your thumb and fingers together, compressing the breast between your thumb and fingers. Do not squeeze hard or pinch. Do not compress the nipple itself (Figure 36).

- Change the position of your thumb and fingers on the breast and repeat the pressing and compressing motion until all parts of the breast have been expressed and the flow of milk slows down. Seeing your breast as the face of a clock, put your thumb and fingers at the 6 o'clock and 12 o'clock positions, then at 1 and 7, 2 and 8, and 3 and 9 (Figure 37).

■ Repeat the procedure on the opposite breast. Express each breast several times until the desired amount of milk has been collected, the flow of milk slows down, or your breasts feel soft. Refrigerate or freeze your milk for later use. See Chapter 20 for storage guidelines.

■ If you need to stop a pumping session before you are done, you can come back to it a short time later.

■ As with breastfeeding, patience and practice are the keys to success.

Figure 36
Hand expression of breastmilk
is economical and easy.
Patience and practice are the
keys to success.

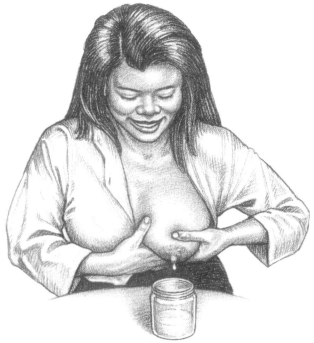

Figure 37
During hand expression, change
the position of your thumb and
fingers on the breast until all
parts of the breast are soft and
the flow of milk slows down.

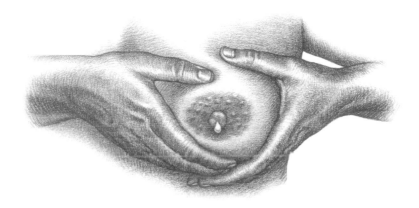

Expressing with a Breast Pump

- Choose a quiet, comfortable place where you will not be disturbed. If necessary take the phone off the hook and lock the door.

- Get organized and gather all of your supplies together. Include a healthy snack and drink for yourself.

- Wash your hands with soap and water and rinse well.

- Put warm water on your breasts. Taking a warm shower or tub bath, using warm washcloths, or soaking the breasts in a pan of warm water works well.

- Gently massage the breasts in a circular pattern using the flat part of your fingers (Figure 22, p. 54).

- Roll your nipple between your thumb and finger. This can cause a let-down reflex and make milk expression easier.

- Relax and think about your baby. This can help milk release and increase the amount of milk obtained. Looking at a picture of your baby, holding something he has worn, listening to music, or listening to a relaxation tape may also be helpful. Plan to do some relaxation exercises at least once a day even if you cannot do them just before pumping.

- Adjust the suction control of the breast pump to the lowest setting. Moisten the pump flange (the cone-shaped part of the pump) with water. Center your nipple in the opening. Follow the directions that come with the pump.

- It may take several minutes for milk to flow. Pump until the flow of milk slows to a drip. If you are pumping both breasts at the same time, rest for several minutes, then repeat once or twice. If you are pumping one breast at a time, you can switch back and forth from breast to breast and do not need to wait. You can slowly increase the suction as long as you are comfortable. With double-pumping you may find that one breast softens before the other and that you still need to single-pump and massage the other breast to relieve the fullness.

- Express each breast several times until the desired amount of milk has been collected or your breasts feel soft. Watch your breasts and the flow of milk, not the clock. Refrigerate or freeze your milk for later use. The collection container that comes with many of the pumps can be used for storage. See Chapter 20 for storage guidelines.

- If you need to stop a pumping session before you are done, you can come back to it a short time later.

- Wash the collection kit after each use in hot, soapy water and rinse well. During work hours, rinse the collection kit in hot water and wash in hot, soapy water when you get home.

- As with breastfeeding, patience and practice are the keys to success.

Choosing a Breast Pump

The best pump is the pump that works for you!

Some mothers rent or purchase a breast pump during their last weeks of pregnancy so that they will be ready for their return to work. But once you hold your baby in your arms, you may find that plans made during pregnancy change. For example, you may end up working fewer hours, and pumping less, than you had planned. So you might want to wait until after your baby is born to choose a breast pump.

Pumps can be rented or purchased from hospitals, pump rental stations, and medical supply companies. Check with your baby's doctor, your lactation consultant, or your nurse for the location nearest your home.

The following information will help you choose a pump that is right for you.

Types of Pumps

The different types of breast pumps available are listed below.

- **Hand pump.** There are many types of hand pumps, including cylinder, squeeze-handle, and rubber-bulb (Figure 12, p. 19). You need two hands to use some hand pumps and only one hand to use others. Many mothers choose hand pumps because they are inexpensive and readily available. While some hand pumps work quite well, others offer poor suction and poor milk removal. Because you cannot control the suction on rubber bulb pumps, nipple damage is more likely to occur, so these pumps should be avoided.

- **Battery-operated pump.** Battery-operated pumps use a small motor and two batteries to generate suction. The type of batteries varies from pump to pump. As the battery power decreases, the strength of the suction decreases as well. Some battery-operated pumps have AC adapters that limit battery use. Some mothers like battery-operated pumps because only one hand is needed to operate the pump. But battery replacement can be very costly if the pump is used often. You can use rechargeable batteries, but they usually produce less suction than alkaline batteries.

- **Semi-automatic electric pump.** Semi-automatic electric pumps create constant suction. To release the suction, you must cover and uncover a small hole in the base of the flange. Too much suction can damage nipples, so care must be taken to release the suction regularly.

■ **Fully automatic electric pump.** Fully automatic electric pumps (Figure 27, p. 73) routinely cycle the amount of suction produced. This limits the risk of nipple damage and increases the amount of milk expressed. In addition, fully automatic electric pumps usually have both single and double collection kits so that you can pump one or both breasts at a time.

Factors to Consider

Factors to consider in choosing a breast pump include:

■ reason for use (to increase your milk supply, to establish a milk supply, to provide an occasional supplement, to feed a preterm infant)

■ frequency of use

■ effectiveness

■ comfort

■ ease of operation

■ ease of cleaning

■ availability

■ durability

■ cost

Features to look for include:

■ pressure range

■ suction control

■ flange size and shape

■ storage capacity

■ backflow protection

Flanges are made out of silicone, soft or hard plastic, or glass. They come in different sizes to fit a variety of nipples and breasts. If necessary an insert can be placed inside the flange to improve the fit.

Many pumps have special parts that fit inside the pump and prevent the flow of expressed milk into the motor or battery case (backflow).

If you plan to pump now and then (once or twice a week), you should consider hand expression, a hand pump, a battery-operated pump, or a semi-automatic electric pump. Hand pumps and battery-operated pumps need to be purchased rather than rented.

If you would like to be able to pump one breast while your baby breastfeeds from the opposite breast, you should consider a squeeze-handle hand pump, a battery-operated pump, or a semi-automatic electric pump. All of these pumps can be operated easily with one hand.

If you plan to pump frequently (one or more times a day) or for many weeks or months, you may want to rent or purchase a fully automatic electric pump.

A fully automatic electric pump usually comes with a double collection kit that lets you pump both breasts at once, saving time and energy (Figure 26, p. 69). In addition, double-pumping increases prolactin levels, which increases milk production.

Most breast pumps are designed to be used by only one person (single-user pumps), but some fully automatic electric pumps can be used by more than one person (multiple-user pumps). Pumps that are used in the hospital (hospital-grade pumps) or are available for rent must be able to be used safely by more than one person. Multiple-user pumps can be cleaned completely to ensure that the breastmilk of one mother does not come into contact with the breastmilk of another mother.

Table 6 on the following page summarizes the best pump to use to meet different goals.

Table 6. Suggestions for Choosing a Breast Pump

GOAL	METHOD OF PUMPING				
	HAND EXPRESSION	HAND PUMP	BATTERY-OPERATED PUMP	SEMI-AUTOMATIC ELECTRIC PUMP	FULLY AUTOMATIC ELECTRIC PUMP
To begin a milk supply					X
To increase a milk supply	X	X	X	X	X
To provide an occasional supplement	X	X	X		
To provide human milk for a hospitalized preterm infant					X
To pump one or two times a week	X	X	X	X	
To pump one or more times a day or for many weeks or months					X
To pump while your baby breastfeeds from the opposite breast		X (squeeze-handle models)	X	X	
To double-pump				X	X

20 Storage of Human Milk

Because storage time and temperature can affect the nutrients in human milk, storage recommendations vary. In the interest of safety, handle your milk the same way you care for other foods: Use containers made for food, store your milk in a cool place, refrigerate it as soon as possible, and freeze it for later use. If you are storing milk for a healthy, full-term baby, follow these simple suggestions:

- Store your milk in any container made for food. Label the container with the date and time. Allow room for expansion if you plan to freeze your milk.

- Place a single serving in each container. More than one container can be thawed if larger amounts are needed. During the first 3 months, babies eat about 2 1/2 ounces per pound each day. An 8-pound baby would eat 2 1/2 ounces x 8, or 20 ounces, per day. Divide the daily intake by the number of feedings and you can estimate the size of a single feeding. Since 20 ounces ÷ 10 feedings = 2 ounces, the mother of an 8-pound baby would want to freeze in 2-ounce servings.

- You can combine small amounts of breastmilk to make a single serving. If you combine fresh milk and frozen milk, chill the fresh milk in the refrigerator first to avoid thawing the frozen layer.

- Recommended storage times vary from study to study. To be safe, store your milk at room temperature (25°C or 77°F) for up to 5 hours, in the refrigerator (4°C or 39°F) for up to 5 days, in the freezer section of a refrigerator/freezer (-5°C or 23°F) for up to 5 months, or in an upright or chest freezer (-20°C or -4°F) for up to 12 months (Figure 38). It's easy to remember storage times, simply count the number of fingers on one hand—five!

■ Human milk stored in the refrigerator or freezer should be placed in the middle of the compartment away from the door to avoid temperature changes. Do not store milk in the refrigerator or freezer door.

■ To thaw, place the unopened container in the refrigerator or in a pan of warm water. Do not thaw or warm any milk for your baby in a microwave oven. A microwave oven destroys live cells and heats the milk unevenly, which increases the risk of burning your baby.

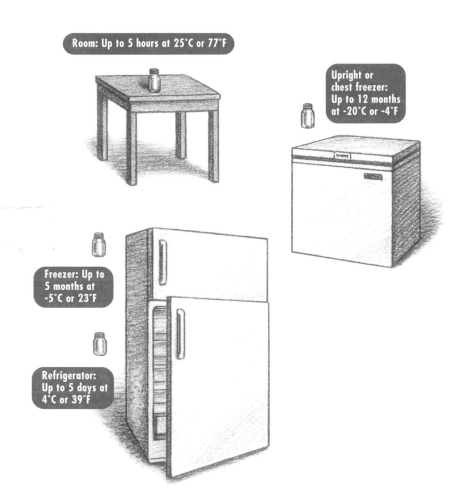

Room: Up to 5 hours at 25°C or 77°F

Upright or chest freezer: Up to 12 months at -20°C or -4°F

Freezer: Up to 5 months at -5°C or 23°F

Refrigerator: Up to 5 days at 4°C or 39°F

Figure 38
Breastmilk storage guidelines for healthy, full-term babies.

- Breastmilk can be served chilled from the refrigerator or at room temperature. No heating is necessary. If your baby prefers milk at room temperature, simply place the unopened container in a pan of warm water for several minutes.

- Milk that has been thawed in the refrigerator should be used within 4 hours once it is removed from the refrigerator or within 24 hours if it is kept in the refrigerator. Milk that has been thawed in a pan of warm water should be used right away or stored in the refrigerator for up to 4 hours.

- Fresh milk left in the feeding container (e.g., bottle or cup) should be stored in the refrigerator and used within 1 hour to complete the feeding. Previously frozen milk left in the feeding container should be discarded.

Table 7. Human Milk Storage Recommendations for Healthy, Full-Term Babies*

HUMAN MILK	ROOM TEMPERATURE (25° C OR 77° F)	REFRIGERATOR (4° C OR 39° F)	FREEZER SECTION (-5° C OR 23° F)	UPRIGHT OR CHEST FREEZER (-20° C OR -4° F)
Fresh	Use within 5 hours	Use within 5 days	Use within 5 months	Use within 12 months
Previously frozen, then thawed in refrigerator	Use within 4 hours	Use within 24 hours	Do not refreeze	Do not refreeze
Previously frozen, then thawed in warm water	Use right away	Use within 4 hours	Do not refreeze	Do not refreeze

* Fresh breastmilk is best for your baby.

21 Weaning Your Baby

How long you breastfeed depends upon your own needs and the needs of your child. Some mothers choose to breastfeed for several weeks, some for several months, and others for several years.

Some babies start to lose interest in breastfeeding between 6 and 12 months when solid foods are introduced, and others are less eager to cuddle and breastfeed once they begin to walk. Occasionally something happens that requires the separation of mother and baby, and makes weaning necessary. But weaning is most often brought about by a mother's need to return to work or school, or by social or cultural pressures.

In many Western cultures, where independence is valued, a baby's first tooth or first step can be seen as a sign that it is time to wean. In reality, the right time to wean is when your child, your partner, or you decide that the time is right. Though family and friends may be eager to offer advice about why, when, and how to wean, only you know what is best for you and your child.

Though even small amounts of breastmilk are valuable, the longer a mother and child breastfeed, the greater the benefits for both. The American Academy of Pediatrics, the World Health Organization, and the United Nations Children's Fund (UNICEF) all recommend exclusive breastfeeding for the first 6 months of life, and continued breastfeeding along with complementary foods for at least 1–2 years.

In spite of these recommendations, mothers in Western cultures who choose to breastfeed beyond the first year are often forced to deal with the disapproval of family and friends. Fortunately, cultural changes are taking place, though slowly. In the meantime, surround yourself with people who support your decision to give your baby the very best!

When Should I Start My Baby on Solid Foods?

There is no magical age at which all babies are suddenly ready for solid foods. Babies grow and develop at their own pace, so it is important to watch your baby for signs indicating that he is ready for solid foods. These signs include the ability to:

- sit up without support
- control his head
- bring food to his mouth
- swallow solid foods without choking

Most babies show an interest in solid foods around 6 months of age and delight in taking food from nearby plates. These early solid food feedings are a learning experience for you and your baby. So don't be surprised to find that most of the food ends up everywhere except your baby's mouth!

How Do I Begin Weaning?

Weaning is a gradual process of babies "taking hold" and mothers "letting go." Weaning begins naturally when solid food or liquids other than breastmilk are introduced, and it continues until breastmilk has been completely replaced by other foods.

The weaning process can last days, weeks, months, or ideally years. Mothers in Western cultures tend to wean earlier than mothers in non-Western cultures, although weaning at a later age is becoming more common. The average age for weaning worldwide is 2–4 years, and in some cultures children breastfeed for 5–7 years.

Weaning is easiest when both mother and child are ready and willing, but more often one or the other leads the way. Given enough time, nearly all children will wean themselves, but culture plays an important role in the decision to wean. Many mothers in Western cultures, where extended breastfeeding is less common, are reluctant to breastfeed beyond the toddler years.

More important than when you wean or why is that the process be gradual. Weaning, particularly if it is sudden, may cause mothers to feel sad or guilty. These feelings are made worse if the baby is unwilling to stop breastfeeding. Feelings of sadness may be due in part to a mother's decrease in prolactin but more importantly to the unexpected end of the breastfeeding relationship.

Some mothers are ready to give up the closeness that breastfeeding provides while others are not. Most mothers have mixed feelings about weaning. These feelings are common and will pass with time, but it may help to talk openly and honestly about your feelings with people you trust. You may also find it helpful to remember that the benefits of breastfeeding continue long after breastfeeding stops.

Suggestions for Weaning Slowly

- Replace one daily breastfeeding at a time with solids or liquids, depending on your baby's age and ability. Choose the breastfeedings in which your baby is the least interested.

- If your baby is under 1 year of age, use iron-fortified formula for replacement feedings. Do not give your baby whole cow's milk. If your child is 1–2 years of age, you can use whole cow's milk. Low-fat or skim milk can be given to children 2 years or older.

- If your baby can sit up, control his head, and bring food to his mouth, he is ready for solid foods. This usually happens at about 6 months of age. Giving solid foods for the first time can be an adventure, so get ready!

- Choose foods that will meet your baby's need for iron. Meats and iron-fortified cereals are suggested.

- Wait 5–7 days before you offer each new food so that you can watch for signs of allergy.

- Place liquids in a bottle or a cup depending on your baby's age and ability. Even newborns can learn to cup-feed, so you may prefer to use a cup and avoid bottles and nipples altogether. If you use a bottle, try different nipple shapes until you find one your baby will accept. A slow-flow nipple may lessen the difference between bottle-feeding and breastfeeding. If you use a cup and your baby is able to sit up and hold the cup by himself, you might want to use a cup with two handles and a snap-on lid to prevent spills.

- Frequently babies refuse foods offered by their mother, so you may need to ask another family member to help with replacement feedings. After many months of breastfeeding, brothers, sisters, and fathers are usually eager for a chance to feed the baby.

- Replace one daily breastfeeding no sooner than every 3–5 days until weaning is complete. Many babies are reluctant to give up the early morning, naptime, and bedtime feedings. If your baby resists, you can continue to breastfeed at those times, but try to shorten the length of feedings.

- Increase cuddling time. Your baby needs to know that separation from the breast does not mean separation from you. Hugs and kisses will let your baby know that your love and affection continue even after breastfeeding stops.

- Distract an active and curious toddler with games, outdoor play, and story-telling.

- Offer foods that appeal to young children, such as finger foods.

- Expect some breastmilk production to continue for many days or even many weeks after weaning is complete.

Suggestions for Sudden Weaning

- Hand express or pump a small amount of milk to relieve fullness and prevent engorgement. A warm washcloth, a warm shower or bath, or soaking the breasts in a pan of warm water can make milk expression easier. Remove only enough milk to relieve fullness and prevent engorgement. The more milk you remove from the breasts, the more milk you will make.

- Put ice on your breasts to relieve pain and reduce swelling. Cold packs, bags of frozen peas wrapped in wet washcloths, or cold, rinsed cabbage leaves work well.

- Wear a snug bra for comfort and support.

- Take acetaminophen or ibuprofen for pain.

22 Common Questions

Will breastfeeding change the size and shape of my breasts?

No. Breastfeeding does not permanently change breast size and shape. Some women find that their breasts get smaller and sag or droop after birth. This can happen whether you choose to breastfeed or not. These changes are due to heredity, age, and weight gain. The more weight you gain during pregnancy, the more your breasts will shrink or sag when the added pounds are lost.

Can I breastfeed and still lose weight?

Yes. You need 500–1,000 calories each day for milk production in addition to the 1,800 calories your body needs. While you can add 500 extra calories to your diet and still lose weight, most mothers produce a good supply of milk without adding extra calories. Fat stored during pregnancy will usually meet your added caloric needs. Frequently mothers find that weight loss has never been easier and work instead to maintain their weight. However, if you are trying to lose unwanted pounds, avoid foods with little or no nutritional value.

Must I follow a special diet while breastfeeding?

No. As long as you eat a variety of foods (breads, fruits, vegetables, dairy products, proteins, and fats), and drink to satisfy your thirst, there is no need to follow a special diet. You can be sure you are getting enough to drink if your urine is clear or pale yellow in color. Sometimes certain foods in a mother's diet make her baby fussy. Milk products, nuts, eggs, wheat, chocolate, and coffee or tea with caffeine may be the cause. Should a certain food make your baby fussy, you may need to limit that food.

Can I smoke while breastfeeding?

Yes and no. Cigarette smoking lowers the fat content of milk and decreases milk production. This may explain why mothers who smoke breastfeed for shorter periods of time. Smoking also increases the risk of sudden infant death syndrome (SIDS). Because the benefits of breastfeeding outweigh the risks of smoking, mothers who smoke are still encouraged to breastfeed. If possible, reduce the number of cigarettes you smoke each day, and avoid smoking in the house or car or near your baby.

Can I drink alcohol while breastfeeding?

Yes and no. Alcohol passes easily into breastmilk. When a mother consumes several drinks each day, the alcohol can affect her baby's motor development (e.g., ability to crawl, walk, grasp, hold). Having even one or two drinks can affect a mother's ability to care for her baby. To reduce the effect of alcohol on you and your baby, drink no more than one or two drinks a week, and avoid breastfeeding for 2 hours after you drink.

Will certain foods change the color of my breastmilk?

Yes. Some mothers have reported orange, green, or black breastmilk when they eat certain foods or take certain medicines. If the color of your breastmilk changes from bluish white (foremilk) or creamy white (hindmilk) to another color, make a list of the foods or medicines you have taken that might be the cause. If the color change continues, contact your doctor, your baby's doctor, or a lactation consultant for help. You can continue to breastfeed as long as your baby shows no signs of illness (vomiting, diarrhea, or fever).

Can I breastfeed if there is blood in my breastmilk?

Yes. Bleeding can occur if there is breast or nipple damage. Your breastmilk can be pink, red, or orange. If your nipples are damaged, put colostrum, breastmilk, or lanolin on the damaged area to aid healing. If the cause of the bleeding is not easily seen or if the bleeding lasts for several days, contact your doctor. You can continue to breastfeed as long as your baby shows no signs of illness (vomiting, diarrhea, or fever). While bleeding is seldom serious, ongoing bleeding can be a sign of breast cancer.

What if I become ill and need medicine?

Most medicines are safe for breastfeeding mothers and babies. Always check with your doctor before taking any medicines, including those available without a prescription (over the counter). Remind your doctor that you are breastfeeding so that she can recommend a medicine that is safe yet effective.

Won't breastfeeding "tie me down"?

Yes and no. In the beginning, when babies are breastfeeding often, breastfeeding can be time-consuming. Once your milk supply is stable (about 6–12 weeks after birth), and your baby is breastfeeding less often, you will find it easier to come and go. If necessary, a substitute feeding can be given using expressed breastmilk or infant formula. The feeding can be given using a cup, hollow-handled medicine spoon, medicine dropper, teaspoon, or bottle, whichever you prefer.

I want to breastfeed, but what if I find it embarrassing?

Some mothers feel embarrassed when they first start to breastfeed; others do not. How you feel will depend on your breastfeeding experience as well as the experience of those around you. Unfortunately, many people see the breast as a sexual object. As a result, many women are uncomfortable handling or exposing their breasts, even for something as natural and wonderful as breastfeeding. Be aware of your own feelings. If necessary, find a private place to breastfeed. Unplug the telephone. Put a small sign on your front door, "Hungry baby, do not disturb." With patience and practice, your confidence in your choice to breastfeed will grow. Remember that experienced mothers can breastfeed discreetly and modestly anywhere (Figure 39).

How can I tell if my baby is getting enough to eat?

The amount of milk taken from the breasts at each feeding cannot be measured. As a result, many mothers worry about whether their baby is getting enough to eat. Remember one important fact about your baby, "Nothing comes out the bottom unless something goes in the top."

The following signs will help to reassure you:

- After day 1, expect at least three stools a day for the next 3 days and at least four stools a day for the next 4 weeks.

  - Your baby's stools will be black and sticky (meconium) on days 1 and 2, green and pasty on days 3 and 4, and yellow, seedy, and runny by day 5.

  - Breastfed babies' stools look like a mix of water, yellow mustard, cottage cheese, and sesame seeds! Expect small, frequent, runny stools with very little solid material. Sometimes all you see in the diaper is a yellow stain the size of your baby's fist.

- After the first 4–6 weeks, expect larger and fewer stools. Many babies have one large stool every 1–5 days, though others continue to have small, frequent stools each day for many months.

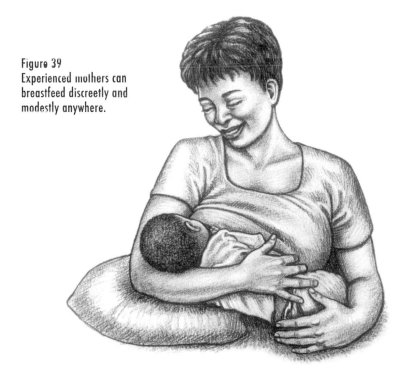

Figure 39
Experienced mothers can breastfeed discreetly and modestly anywhere.

- Expect your baby to have clear or pale yellow urine and at least six wet diapers a day by day 5. Many parents find it hard to tell if a disposable diaper is wet because they hold liquid so well. To check for wetness, place several sheets of toilet paper inside the diaper when a new diaper is used.

- While wet diapers are important, a decrease in the number of stools is the first sign that your baby may not be getting enough to eat (see Table 8).

Do I need to give my baby vitamin and mineral supplements?

Yes and no. If you have a healthy, full-term baby, your milk provides nearly all the vitamins, minerals (iron and fluoride), and nutrients your baby needs for the first 6 months of life. There are two exceptions, vitamins K and D. Vitamin K is given right after birth to prevent bleeding. The main source of vitamin D is the sun, but sunlight is hard to measure. Because too much sunlight can be harmful, doctors recommend a supplement of 200 IU of vitamin D each day beginning by 2 months of age. Babies store enough iron in their livers during the last weeks of pregnancy to meet their iron needs for about 6 months. After 6 months, iron-fortified solid foods like meats are recommended.

If I breastfeed, can I give my baby a pacifier?

Yes and no. Pacifiers can interfere with your baby's suckling pattern, decrease your milk supply, increase the risk of ear infections, and lead to early weaning. But some studies show that pacifiers may reduce the risk of SIDS. During the early weeks, when you and your baby are learning to breastfeed, pacifiers should be avoided. After your baby is breastfeeding well (4–6 weeks after birth) and gaining weight (4–8 ounces a week), you can offer a pacifier. Because some babies want to suck beyond their need to eat, some mothers may find a pacifier helpful. However, many breastfed babies prefer to suck on their fists, thumbs, or fingers and often refuse pacifiers.

Can I sleep with my baby?

Yes and no. When babies are within reach, nighttime feedings are easier, mothers get more sleep, and babies have less risk of sudden infant death syndrome (SIDS). Research shows that babies often sleep

Table 8. Important Signs That Every Breastfeeding Parent Should Know

SIGNS THAT YOUR BABY IS WELL FED*	SIGNS THAT YOUR BABY MAY NOT BE GETTING ENOUGH TO EAT*
Your baby is alert and active.	Your baby is unusually sleepy.
Your baby is happy and satisfied after breastfeeding.	Your baby is restless and fussy after breastfeeding.
Your baby breastfeeds at least 8 times in each 24 hours.	Your baby breastfeeds fewer than 8 times in each 24 hours.
You hear or see your baby swallow when he breastfeeds.	You can't hear or see your baby swallow when he breastfeeds.
Your baby loses less than 7% of his birth weight during the first 5 days.	Your baby loses more than 7% of his birth weight during the first 5 days.
Your baby begins to gain weight after day 5 and is back to his birth weight by 10 days of age.	Your baby continues to lose weight after day 5 and is below his birth weight at 10 days of age.
Your baby gains 4–8 ounces each week after the first week.	Your baby gains less than 4 ounces each week after the first week.
Your baby has 3 or more stools** a day after day 1, increasing to 4 or more stools a day by day 5.	Your baby has less than 3 stools** a day after day 1.
Your baby's stool changes from black to yellow by day 5.	Your baby's stool is still black or green on day 5.
Your baby has clear or pale yellow urine and 6 or more wet diapers a day by day 5.	Your baby has red or dark yellow urine and less than 6 wet diapers a day by day 5.

* If you see signs that your baby is not getting enough to eat, call your baby's health care provider right away.
** A stool is a stain the size of your baby's fist or at least 1 teaspoon of solid material.

in more than one place, including car seats, cribs, cots, bassinets, co-sleepers (baby beds that attach to the side of adult beds), and adult beds. While some sleep areas are safe, others are not. Certain conditions and behaviors can make a safe area an unsafe one. The following suggestions will help you keep your baby safe.

- Place your baby on his back. Do not put your baby on his tummy or side.

- Use a lightweight cover. Do not use comforters, duvets, quilts, or pillows.

- Dress your baby in a single layer of clothing. Do not let your baby get too hot.

- Place your baby on a firm mattress. Do not place your baby on a waterbed, sofa, or chair.

- Do not place your baby alone in an adult bed.

- Do not place your baby in an adult bed with older children.

- Parents should not sleep with their baby if they are overly tired.

- Parents who smoke should not sleep with their baby.

- Parents should not sleep with their baby if they have used alcohol or drugs.

- Parents who are very overweight should not sleep with their baby.

If you have questions about co-sleeping, talk with your baby's health care provider.

If my baby has colic, can I still breastfeed?

Yes. Colic—long periods of fussing and crying each day for no clear reason—occurs in 10–20 percent of newborns. Colic occurs in formula-fed babies as well as in breastfed babies. The symptoms usually appear 2–6 weeks after birth and disappear by 12–16 weeks of age. The cause of colic is unclear. Occasionally overfeeding or something in the infant's or the mother's diet can cause fussiness. Often no cause is found.

If you have a very fussy baby, offer one breast at each feeding. The result will be a low-volume, low-sugar, high-fat meal rather than a high-volume, high-sugar, low-fat meal. In addition, avoid giving your baby formula containing cow's milk, and avoid consuming milk products, eggs, nuts, and wheat yourself (see "Breastfeeding a Baby with a Family History of Allergic Disease," p. 106).

Constant sounds or vibrations from a vacuum cleaner, clothes dryer, car engine, or untuned television may soothe a fussy baby. A warm compress on the abdomen can also be helpful. A warm tub bath, a warm washcloth, or a warm water bottle works well. While colic seldom lasts more than 16 weeks, it can seem like 16 years! A mother unable to calm her baby feels guilty. A father unable to calm his partner feels helpless. If the fussiness continues, medicine can be helpful. You will need to call your baby's doctor for a prescription.

Weaning is seldom necessary. Frequently, the use of infant formula makes the symptoms worse. As the infant grows and the intestinal tract matures, the symptoms will improve. While infants in some cultures typically cry 2–3 hours a day, in cultures where babies are carried in slings for much of the day, colic is rarely seen.

I tried to breastfeed my first baby, but I was unable to produce enough milk. How can I keep this from happening again?

Nearly every mother worries about her ability to produce enough milk. Some women have a small number of milk-producing cells (alveoli); however, this is rare. When a mother's milk supply or a baby's weight gain is low, it is usually the result of too little knowledge or too little support. The following suggestions will help you build and keep a good milk supply:

- Breastfeed whenever your baby seems fussy or hungry. During the early weeks, expect to breastfeed 8–12 times in each 24 hours or every 1–3 hours during the day and every 2–3 hours at night. Sometimes a sleepy baby will not ask to eat often enough. Therefore, during the first 4 weeks, keep your baby with you day and night. Watch for early signs of hunger or light sleep such as squirming, rapid eye movements, sucking sounds, hand-to-mouth movements, yawning, or coughing, and offer the breast at those times.

- Breastfeed as long as your baby wishes on the first breast before offering the second breast. If your baby falls asleep while breast-feeding and the first breast is still firm and full, break the suction, burp him, wake him, and put him back on the first breast.

- Offer both breasts at every feeding. However, do not be concerned if your baby seems satisfied with one breast. Remember that each breast can provide a full meal. It is more important that your baby breastfeed well on one breast than that he breastfeed on both breasts.

- Begin each feeding on the breast offered last.

- Avoid the use of water or formula supplements during the first 4 weeks. Supplements can interfere with your baby's suckling pattern and limit breastmilk production.

- Drink to satisfy your thirst. Clear or pale yellow urine will let you know you are getting enough to drink. Water and unsweetened fruit juices are suggested. It is not necessary to drink milk to make milk. Mothers who drink lots of milk or eat lots of milk products can have fussy babies.

- Eat a balanced diet.

- Get plenty of rest. Nap when your baby naps.

- Should problems occur, get help from people trained to help breast-feeding mothers.

How much weight should my baby gain in the beginning?

Your baby should lose no more than 7 percent of his birth weight during the first 5 days and should regain that weight by day 10. After the first 5 days, your baby should gain 4–8 ounces a week. Sometimes a baby will gain slowly. However, breastfeeding patterns should be carefully reviewed, so you can be sure that your baby is getting enough to eat.

Babies often double their birth weight by 4–6 months of age and triple their birth weight by 1 year of age.

I plan to give my baby a substitute feeding using expressed breastmilk. How much milk will I need to express for a feeding?

A healthy, full-term baby needs about 2 1/2 ounces per pound each day (see "Estimate the size of a single serving during the first 3 months," p. 117). For example, a 10-pound baby would require 2 1/2 x 10, or 25 ounces, a day. If the baby breastfeeds every 2–3 hours, or 10 times a day, and eats 25 ounces a day, then he eats about 2 1/2 ounces at each feeding. To be on the safe side, express 4–6 ounces of breast-milk and store the milk in 2- to 3-ounce servings to avoid waste. You can use more than one serving if necessary.

Some mothers prefer to substitute with infant formula. Ask your baby's doctor for a recommendation.

Will breastfeeding affect my sex life?

Some mothers have less desire for sex due to tiredness, fear of pregnancy, or fear of pain. Others find that breastfeeding alone provides enough touching and holding to satisfy their sexual needs. Still others are eager to have sex. Discuss your feelings openly with your partner.

Many breastfeeding mothers have dryness in the vagina (birth canal) that can cause pain during intercourse (sex). A water soluble lubricant such as K-Y Jelly may be helpful. Put a small amount around the opening of the vagina before having sex.

When you have sex, you may have a climax or orgasm. Orgasm causes the release of oxytocin from the brain. Oxytocin causes the release of milk from the breasts. Some fathers feel like they have to come to bed thirsty or carry an umbrella! To limit the risk of leakage during sex, breastfeed your baby before making love.

If I breastfeed, can I still get pregnant?

Yes and no. You can achieve natural child spacing if you breastfeed fully (exclusively or almost exclusively). However, if your breastfeeding schedule or routine limits the frequency or length of breastfeedings or includes frequent use of breastmilk substitutes, pregnancy is more likely.

Ovulation (egg release) and menstruation (monthly bleeding) may not occur while you are breastfeeding, especially during the first 6-12 weeks. However, most women resume ovulation and menstruation while breastfeeding. Ovulation can occur before menstruation, therefore, do not assume that you are protected (safe) before your first menstrual period.

If pregnancy is not desired, a safe method of birth control is suggested. Your choices include cervical cap, female condom, diaphragm, intrauterine device, tubal ligation, male condom, vasectomy, and spermicidal cream, foam, or jelly. Birth control pills that contain estrogen

and progesterone (combination pills) are not recommended (Figure 1,
p. 5). However, birth control pills (minipills), implants (Implanon,
Norplant), or injections (Depo-Provera) that contain only progesterone
are thought to be safe (see p. 5). Discuss the choices with your health
care provider.

If I become pregnant, can I still breastfeed?

Yes and no. Many mothers continue to breastfeed during pregnancy
and have two babies or a baby and a child at the breast after birth.
This is called tandem nursing. To meet the needs of two growing
babies, you will need to eat a balanced diet that includes extra calories,
drink to satisfy your thirst, and nap when the babies nap. As long as
the younger baby is fully breastfed and the older baby is taking some
solid foods, you should breastfeed the younger baby first.

During pregnancy, a mother's breasts and nipples can become tender,
and the volume and content of her breastmilk change. When breastmilk volume decreases, sodium and protein increase, and lactose and
glucose (sugars) decrease, making the milk look and taste more like
colostrum. Sometimes the older baby or child loses interest in the
breast (child-led weaning), or breast tenderness, common during pregnancy, makes breastfeeding painful, and weaning occurs (mother-led
weaning).

Breastfeeding can cause uterine contractions, but there is no evidence
to suggest that the developing fetus (unborn baby) is at risk. However,
if you have a history of premature labor or vaginal bleeding during
pregnancy, your doctor or midwife may suggest that you wean (see
"Weaning Your Baby," p. 152).

Do I need to stop breastfeeding when my baby's teeth come in?

No. You do not need to wean when your baby's teeth come in. Biting
can occur at the end of a feeding, when your baby is no longer hungry,
but playful. Simply remove your baby from the breast with a firm "no."
If your baby is still hungry, offer the breast again. If the biting continues, remove your baby from the breast for several minutes. Your baby
will soon learn that biting brings an end to breastfeeding, and the biting will stop.

How long should I breastfeed?

You should breastfeed until you or your baby decides that it is time to stop. This may be several weeks, several months, or several years. Doctors recommend breastfeeding alone for the first 6 months. Then solid foods should gradually be introduced, reducing the need for human milk. However, human milk or infant formula is necessary during the first year of life. Many women choose to breastfeed until their baby can be weaned easily to solid foods and a cup (12–24 months). Continuing to breastfeed avoids the added cost of bottles and formula.

What are growth spurts?

Growth spurts or frequency days often occur around 3 weeks, 6 weeks, 3 months, and 6 months. However, growth spurts can occur at any time. Your baby may be fussy and restless and want to breast-

Figure 40
Doctors recommend
breastfeeding alone for
the first 6 months.

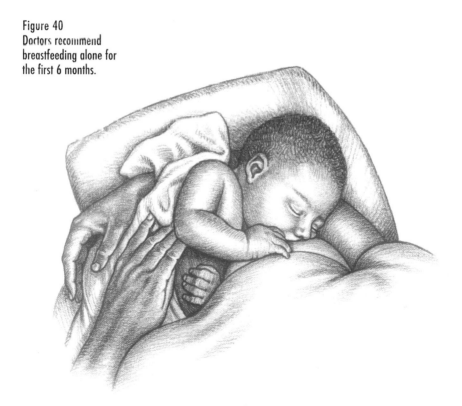

feed all the time. Well-meaning but inexperienced friends and relatives may suggest that "your milk isn't rich enough," that "you're not making enough milk," that "solid foods or a formula supplement is necessary," or that "it is time to stop breastfeeding." After 2–3 days of frequent breastfeedings, your milk supply will catch up with the increased demand, and the length and frequency of breastfeedings will decrease.

What are nursing strikes?

A nursing strike occurs when a baby suddenly refuses to breastfeed. A strike can last for several feedings or several days. Sometimes the cause is easily identified, such as teething, fever, ear infection, stuffy nose (cold), constipation, or diarrhea. Occasionally, menstruation (monthly bleeding) or something in your diet will change the taste of your milk. Deodorant, perfume, or powder placed on the mother's skin can be the cause of the strike. Frequently no cause is found.

Until the strike ends, you will need to hand express or pump to relieve fullness and maintain your milk supply. Continue to offer the breast. However, do not insist if your baby refuses. Give expressed breastmilk by teaspoon, eye dropper, hollow-handled medicine spoon, or cup until breastfeeding resumes. Be patient and relax. Watch for early signs of hunger and offer the breast at those times. Limit noise and distractions during feedings. Give your baby undivided attention. Nursing strikes seldom lead to weaning. With time, your baby will return to the breast.

Can I breastfeed if I am HIV positive?

The Centers for Disease Control and Prevention (CDC) and the World Health Organization (WHO) recommend that HIV-positive women not breastfeed, as long as they live in countries where clean, safe supplies (water, formula, bottles, and nipples) are available for feeding their babies. However, in countries where the risk of death during the first year of life from diarrhea and other infections is high (greater than 50 percent), breastfeeding is encouraged even among HIV-positive women. Heat treatment of expressed breastmilk, exclusive breastfeeding, and the use of antiviral medicine during pregnancy and after birth may reduce the risk of mother-to-child transmission.

Can I breastfeed if I use illegal drugs?

No. Women who are chemically dependent and actively abusing drugs should not breastfeed. However, recovering drug users who remain drug-free can breastfeed. Close follow-up is important for both you and your baby.

Can I exercise if I am breastfeeding?

Yes. Moderate exercise does not affect the amount of milk produced or the taste of the milk.

23 Congratulations, You're a Parent!

You may think that once your baby is born the hard part will be over. But the truth is that the hard part will just be beginning. A typical labor and birth can last up to 18 hours, but parenting lasts 18 (or more) years! Unfortunately, nothing can prepare you fully for the days and weeks to come. While reading books on baby care can be helpful, there is no substitute for on-the-job training. So take a deep breath and try to relax. You're about to become a parent.

Many parents are surprised to find that the excitement and anticipation they felt during pregnancy are quickly replaced by fear and frustration. With 4 hours of uninterrupted sleep a distant memory, even the most confident parents begin to doubt their ability to care for their baby.

"I can do this."

"Can I do this?"

"I can't do this!"

"I have to do this."

"How can I do this?"

In the beginning you will want to concentrate on learning how to feed, hold, and calm your baby. As your ability to care for your baby grows, you will have more time for other tasks.

In some cultures, a new mother is expected to do everything by herself. In other cultures, family members come and stay for weeks or even months to care for the mother while she cares for her baby. Either way, babies require a lot of work.

Don't Expect Everything to be Perfect

Parents today are under tremendous pressure to be perfect. But many parents find breastfeeding much more difficult than they thought it would be. Though some mothers and babies—the lucky few—know just what to do, most need to learn. So don't feel that you have to be an expert from the start. It may take several days or weeks for you and your baby to master the art of breastfeeding.

"I thought breastfeeding was supposed to be natural."

"I felt like a failure when I couldn't get my baby to latch on to my breast."

"My baby slept all the time. I couldn't get him awake to breastfeed."

"I was afraid to tell my friends that I had stopped breastfeeding."

If you have difficulty breastfeeding, you will find it reassuring to know that there is a solution to nearly every problem. Keep this book handy and refer to it as needed. Grandmothers, mothers, sisters, aunts, and friends may be eager to offer advice, but their knowledge of breast-feeding may be limited. So be sure to get help from someone trained to help breastfeeding mothers.

The more breastmilk your baby receives, the greater the health bene-fits. Health professional organizations recommend exclusive breast-feeding for the first 6 months, and continued breastfeeding for at least 1 year. If you are unable to breastfeed exclusively, you and your baby will still benefit from whatever amount of breastmilk you provide and from the closeness that comes with breastfeeding.

Some mothers, despite every effort, are unable to breastfeed their babies. Fortunately, these situations are rare. If you happen to be a mother who cannot breastfeed, infant formula can provide the basic nutrients your baby needs to grow.

Expect the Unexpected

No amount of planning can prepare you for the day when you are still in your nightgown at 3:00 in the afternoon, when your baby wants to breastfeed every hour, when a clean house and home-cooked meals are memories of a former life, and when sleep is more appealing than sex!

Parenting is the most important job you will ever hold, yet it is the job for which you will have the least training. You will be required to work 24 hours a day, 7 days a week, 52 weeks a year—including weekends, nights, and holidays. There will be no benefits package—no pension plan, no paid vacation, no sick leave. There won't even be a salary. The only compensation you will receive will be a smile, a laugh, a hug, a first word, a first step, a first tooth. And looking back in years to come, with no reservations or hesitation, you would do it all again!

Cherish every moment.

What Does That Word Mean?

Alveoli: Alveoli are grape-like clusters of cells inside the breast that produce milk.

Antibodies: Antibodies are special proteins that protect you and your baby from infection.

Areola: The areola is the darker (pigmented) part of the breast around the nipple.

Colostrum: Colostrum is the first milk your breasts make. It can be thick and yellow or clear and runny. Colostrum is produced during the last weeks of pregnancy and the first days after birth.

Estrogen: Estrogen is a hormone produced by the placenta. It inhibits the release of prolactin and the production of milk during pregnancy.

Foremilk: Foremilk is obtained at the start of a breastfeeding. It is low in protein, fat, and calories, giving it a thin, runny appearance.

Hindmilk: Hindmilk is obtained near the end of a breastfeeding. It is high in protein, fat, and calories, giving it a thick, creamy appearance.

Lactation: Lactation is the period of milk production.

Let-down or milk-ejection reflex: When your baby breastfeeds (suckles), a let-down, or milk-ejection, reflex occurs. Milk flows from the milk-producing cells (alveoli) into the milk ducts, where it is available to your baby.

Meconium: Meconium is a black, sticky material found in the lower bowel of newborns.

Milk ducts: Milk ducts are small tubes that carry milk from the milk-producing cells (alveoli) to the openings in the nipple.

Montgomery's glands: Montgomery's glands are small, pimple-like bumps in the darker part of the breast (areola) around the nipple.

Oxytocin: Oxytocin is a hormone that causes the muscles around the milk-producing cells (alveoli) to contract.

Pituitary gland: The pituitary gland is a small group of cells attached to the base of the brain. The pituitary gland produces hormones that regulate growth, reproduction, and lactation.

Placenta: The placenta (afterbirth) is an organ inside the uterus that transfers nutrients from mother to baby during pregnancy.

Progesterone: Progesterone is a hormone produced by the placenta. It inhibits the release of prolactin and the production of milk during pregnancy.

Prolactin: Prolactin is a hormone that causes the milk-producing cells (alveoli) to make milk.

Uterus: The uterus is a hollow, muscular organ in which babies develop and grow during pregnancy.

Vagina: The vagina (birth canal) is the passageway that the baby goes through during birth.

Weaning: Weaning is the replacement of breastmilk with other foods or liquids. When your baby no longer receives breastmilk, weaning is complete.

Where Can I Find Help?

To find an International Board Certified Lactation Consultant (IBCLC)* in your area, contact:

International Lactation Consultant Association
1500 Sunday Drive, Suite 102
Raleigh, NC 27607
Tel: (919) 861-5577
Fax: (919) 787-4916
E-mail: info@ilca.org
Website: ilca.org

To find a La Leche League Leader** in your area, contact:

La Leche League International
1400 North Meacham Road
Schaumburg, IL 60168-4079
Tel: (800) 525-3243
Fax: (847) 519-0035
E-mail: LLLHQ@llli.org
Website: lalecheleague.org

---

* An International Board Certified Lactation Consultant is a health care provider with special skills in lactation and breastfeeding management. To become an IBCLC, an individual must pass an independent examination administered by the International Board of Lactation Consultant Examiners (IBLCE).

** A La Leche League Leader is an experienced mother who has breastfed her own children and who has been trained by La Leche League International to answer your questions.

Index

About the Author

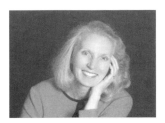

Amy Spangler, MN, RN, IBCLC, is a wife, mother, nurse, lactation consultant, educator, and author. She earned her bachelor's degree in nursing from the Ohio State University and her master's degree in maternal and infant health from the University of Florida. Amy is a registered nurse, an International Board Certified Lactation Consultant, a former president of the International Lactation Consultant Association, and a former chair of the United States Breastfeeding Committee. Amy has worked with mothers, babies, and families for over 30 years. She and her husband live in Atlanta, Georgia, and have two sons.

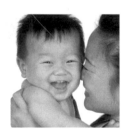

For more information about our products, please contact:

Amy's Babies
P.O. Box 501046
Atlanta, GA 31150-1046
Tel: (770) 913-9332
Fax: (770) 913-0822
E-mail: amyspangler@amysbabies.com
Website: amysbabies.com